Street Saints of Compassion

**The wanton destruction of the worlds largest
Emergency Medical Service
By
*FDNY***

Jim Schrang

Copyright © 2007 by Jim Schrang

ISBN 978-0-7414-4421-9

Published by:

INFI∞ITY
PUBLISHING.COM

1094 New DeHaven Street, Suite 100
West Conshohocken, PA 19428-2713
Info@buybooksontheweb.com
www.buybooksontheweb.com
Toll-free (877) BUY BOOK
Local Phone (610) 941-9999
Fax (610) 941-9959

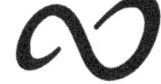

Printed in the United States of America

Published October 2012

You've heard of RAMBO,...
you've heard of PSYCHO,...
GET READY FOR

Jimbo!

Burp!!

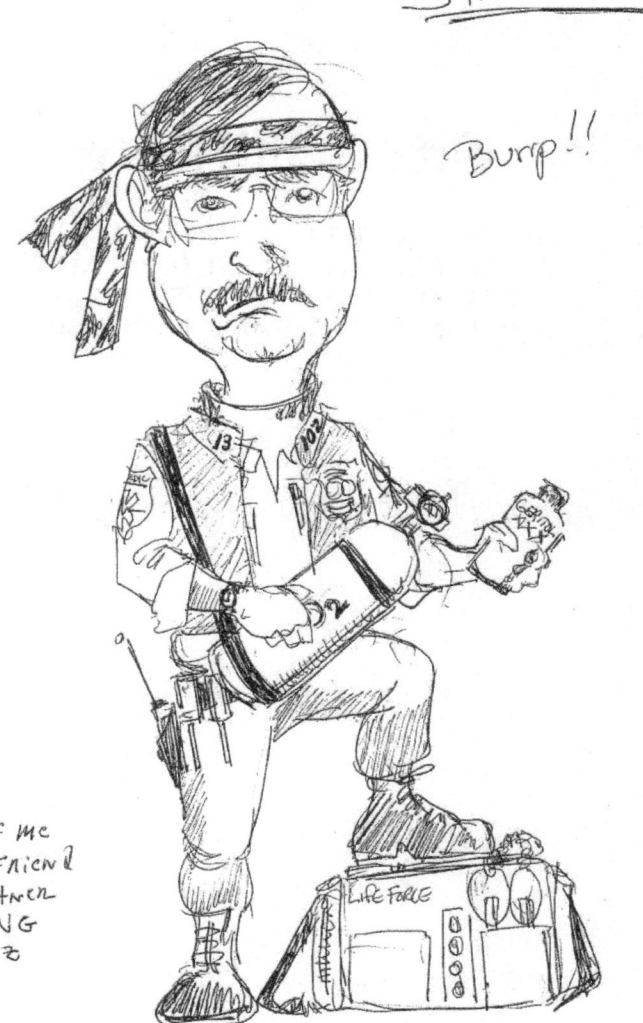

DRAWN OF ME
by my FRIEND
And pARTNER
JACK NG
OF 10♥

Gift Certificate

**THANK YOU FOR CALLING 911, AGAIN !
YOUR CONSTANT ABUSE OF 911 NOW
ENTITLES YOU TO A FREE LETHAL
INJECTON AT ANY EMERGENCY ROOM.**

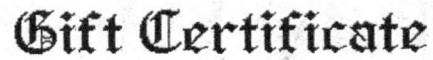

JAMES KERR, EXECUTIVE DIRECTOR

Dedication

"Currahee" is a Native American word meaning "stand alone." It was my battalion logo when I was an army paratrooper with the 101st Airborne Division, "Screaming Eagles," in Vietnam and Cambodia.

This book is bittersweet for not only does it open wounds that need to be cleaned, but it also rejoices at the caliber of people that were the heart of NYC EMS and later FDNY EMS before I put my papers in. The book is dedicated to *three* especially beloved females. All walked this path we call life in obscurity, known for the most part to only family and friends. The first remarkable woman was a very young Native American girl named Sakakawea who was born of the Shoshoni and enslaved by the Hidatsa nations. This young lady courageously led Lewis and Clark across a dangerous new wilderness known as America. Diary excerpts reflect their unyielding respect for this girl's profound knowledge, skills, bravery, calmness under extremely dangerous conditions and always friendly gentle spirit. The way she passed into eternity is contested. Some say by fever at the age of 24 years old, others by a gunshot at the age of 81. In both stories she never complained.

So too the following girls led us by their very presence with all the graceful qualities of Sakakawea's unselfish, pioneering spirit of love. I have no doubt Sacagawea surely calls them *her* American daughters.

Both were different, yet both wore an EMT patch on their shoulder. Both graced each of us with their love and will continue to be with my brothers and sisters in the dark, lonely hours as they continue the Dance of Life.

Tracy Allen Lee, who on September 24, 1989 became the first NYC EMS professional to die of AIDS contracted while performing her duties. Bubbly, funny, always caring, Tracy's smile still warms the hearts of all she blessed with her presence. A fragile, loving healer harassed upon her deathbed by "Law and Order" Mayor Rudolph Giuliani and FDNY.

Yamel Merino, a young single mother, on that fateful day when war was declared against the United States of America, gave her all. When the fireball of man's insane hatred consumed all, creating a living hell on earth, FDNY EMS Command evaporated. In this dire, chaotic moment in history, individual EMS crewmembers, not pundits or political "experts," bonded in blood, sweat, and tears and stood together. A woman petrified by burning bodies jumping to their death, having a young son to live for, still believed in love and softly stepped into hell. Yamel gave up the physical life for something all healers know is greater than hatred, or life itself: eternal love. For in the end, only love remains; Yamel knew this and lived it.

In the end, through our tears we would know—not believe, _but know_—that love outshined the insanity of hatred that murdered thousands that day and continues to. I think it is fitting that in a nation, and a world, that places so much emphasis on the illusion of ego centered male machismo, this book is dedicated to two seemingly obscure young minority women, united by one young Native American.

The paramedics and emergency medical technicians of New York City are true American "Currahees," and much richer for these precious American warrior healers who led the way. The stories within are also dedicated to the volunteer EMS units both from NY and NJ and from surrounding States who responded in on 9-11. FDNY EMS gave them radios and told them to "answer calls." They never were given even a map, yet accomplished their mission as EMS crews' worldwide do 24x7 with compassion and distinction.

Finally, this is dedicated to the volunteer firefighters who responded only to be thrown off the "pile" for "security reasons" when the President arrived. The reality was FDNY ego had a photo op they just couldn't afford to miss, or mess up with volunteers.

Thus to the volunteer EMS and firefighters I say what FDNY never did, thank you. This is your story since, just as Sakakawea, Tracy and Yamel taught both in life and death, we are but one family.

Jim Schrang, FDNY Paramedic (Retired)

CONTENTS

List of abbreviations

ACR (Ambulance Call Report)
ALS (Advanced Life Support)
AMS (Altered Mental Status)
ANFO (Ammonium Nitrate/Fuel Oil) Bomb
APE (Acute Pulmonary Edema)
BBP (Blood-borne Pathogens)
BHS (Bureau of Health Services)
BITS (Bureau of Investigation and Trials)
BLS (EMT)
BUS Ambulance as it is called in New York City
BVM (Bag Valve Mask)
CC (Civilian Complaint)
CCU (Civilian Complaint Unit)
CD (Command Discipline)
CFR (Certified First Responders)
CFRD (Certified First Responder; D defibrillator)
CHF (Congestive Heart Failure)
Circling the Drain: Patient about to die
CISM (Critical Incident Stress Management
CO (Commanding Officer)
CPR (Cardiopulmonary Resuscitation)
DC (Deputy Chief)
DOI (Department of Investigation)
DOT (Department of Traffic)

EDP (Every Day Person)

EDP (Extremely Disturbed People or Every Day Person)

EEO (Equal Employment & Opportunity)

EFP (Explosively Formed Projectiles)

ELI (Emergency Locator Indicator)

EMS (Emergency Medical Service)

EMTs (Emergency Medical Technicians)

Escape mask/hood: Used to evacuate scene of chemical incident good for only 5-30 minutes at most.

ESU (NYPD Emergency Service Unit)

ETA (Estimated Time of Arrival)

FDNY (Fire Department New York)

FDI (Fire Department Institute)

FEMA (Federal Emergency Management Agency)

FUBAR (Fucked Up Beyond Any Repair)

HAZMAT (Hazardous Materials)

Hatzolah (Jewish volunteers)

ICU (Intensive Care Unit)

IED (Improvised Explosive Device)

ISU (Inspectional Service Unit)

KDT (Onboard Computer System)

Level A suit: Highest protection, encapsulated suit with no external openings, gas tight, cumbersome to ware & work in.

Level B suit: Next grade lower in protection with external oxygen air supply.

Level C suit: Lowest form of protective wear. Charcoal suit, not gas tight, & worn with gas mask. Employed by U.S. troops in Chemical, Biological attack.

LODI (Line of Duty Injuries)

MAST (Military Anti-Shock Trousers)

MCI (Mass Casualty Incidents)

MERV (Manned Emergency Response Vehicle)

MTA (Mass Transit Administration)

MOP & GLOW (Haz-Mat Team)

Mr. Murphy & Murphy (What can go wrong will)

MVO (Motor Vehicle Operator)

MVA (Motor Vehicle Accident)

NYC EMS (New York City Emergency Medical Services)

NYPD (New York Police Department)

OPG (Operating Procedure Guide)

PESH (Public Employee Safety and Health Bureau)

PRU (Paramedic Response Units)

RCC (Resources Coordination Center)

Ring of Concern: Reference by Paramedics and EMT's concerning FDNY firefighters standing around patient providing no care, just the stare.

SOD (Special Operations Division)

SRO (Single Room Occupancy)

Stare of Care: See Ring of Concern

SNAFU (Situation Normal All Fucked Up)

Toxic Brain Syndrome: Too much FDNY ego with not enough oxygen to the remaining brain cells.

UFOA (Uniform Fire Officers Association)

VBED (Vehicle Bomb Explosive Device)

Preface

Did FDNY pass money to the publisher to kill this book originally?

FDNYEMSWEBSITE@AOL.COM
6/4/2005 3:08:04 PM

I am very interested in it. I looked up the listings on Amazon.com and Barns and Noble and I loved every word written in the preview. **EMS and FDNY Brass are very upset with you over the book and you have so many people worried over this that there will be a meeting Monday at 9 Metrotech on how to deal with any fallout from the book.** I love it and I will support the book by giving it a link and a glowing review on my page. With 186,000 readers every month it will get you a few sales.

For what it's worth I am very proud of you and the work that you have done. You are my hero.

FDNYEMSWEBSITE@AOL.COM
6/4/2005 10:01:06 PM

Great news let me know the second it hits amazon.com because I will link it so you can get sales. Any promo work that you are doing I can help by giving it good publicity if you like. I am so happy that this is happening. This is just great. Anything you need on the WWW end just ask and I will help.

I GOT THE BOOK! Jim, I must say it looks terrific. I can't wait to get started reading and I may even have to start before I go on vacation. Your explanation below really clears up a lot for me and I am glad to hear that you see the FTG thing the way you do. Yep... time to let the Lawyer take over, and besides topless joints and cocktails, I am sure there are a million other things you'd rather be doing than dealing with Joel or Larry. **Clearly they don't scare you**, and **obviously I am not going to quit communication with you because and email from Larry told you to.** I can be friends with whom ever I want... client of FTG or not.

All my best,
Nicole

***

Nicole forwarded this to me.

From: "maria NA" <maria-tfg@hotmail.com>
To: bradpan@verizon.net
Subject: IMPORTANT NOTICE...From The Floating Gallery
Date: Wed, 20 Jul 2005 17:06:01 -0400

Dear Client:

It has come to our attention that charges of fraud and theft have been brought against Eric Coates, a one-time subcontractor of The Floating Gallery.

We have been notified that there is a possible investigation by The New York State Attorney General's Office underway into the dealings that Mr. Coates has allegedly been engaged in.

The Floating Gallery has severed all ties with Eric Coates and is also looking into its own lawsuit against Mr. Coates for defamation and tortious interference with contract, including libel, slander and theft of services.

Mr. Coates is not and never was an employee of The Floating Gallery or Advanced-Self-Publishing-Book.com. Mr. Coates was a subcontractor used by a number of publishing firms, including ours. Mr. Coates was only contracted for typesetting work by The Floating Gallery. To all our clients, please be rest assured that all your typesetting work is safely with us. We regret any inconvenience.

If Mr. Coates contacts you whether by phone, mail or E-mail, please let us know immediately. **We will forward that information to the proper authorities.**

But whatever you do, we strongly urge you NOT to pay him any money for any reason.

If you have any questions, please call or e-mail The Floating Gallery.

Sincerely,

Joel Hochman
Laurence Leichman
The Floating Gallery

***

Tee Time Girl   7/28/2005 11:51:29 PM

Your book is not what I normally pick up, but I can't seem to put it down. You are a riot to read. I love your sense of humor and your style is so "in your face", I love it. I know if I were choosing sides in life, I would definitely want you on

my side. Hey, what do you know? We are playing life and we do get to choose who we want on our teams!!! Tag. I'll talk to you more when I get back from Vacation.
Nicole

Note: "We will forward that information to the proper authorities." Interestingly they <u>never did</u> contact the authorities, <u>never did pay me</u> for copies sold under Hudson Books or subsidiary companies. Gee does that make them thieves? Mr. Lawerence Leichman tried to intimidate me with, "You don't know who you are dealing with! This is your last chance!" Evidently this idiot has been watching too many Godfather movies, learning nothing. First, you don't leave threats on voicemail, duh. Next, if you are a man, make the statement up close and personal. Finally, a criminal background of Lawerence Leichman, Joel Hochman, Eric Coates and Hudson Books proved to be extremely interesting...

So did <u>FDNY pass money to these people</u> to kill my book? Well I don't know and I would never say that. I'll let you gentle readers decide after reading this *updated* version. Oh, and since FDNY was afraid of this book which was originally **Civilian Warriors, Civilian Healers** 'Conspiracies, Rape, and Cover-Ups in the Firehouse' then they should be very afraid of this updated version **Street Saints of Compassion** 'FDNY's destruction of NYC EMS and petrified of it's companion book **FDNY Illusion of Security**. If they annoy me I still have more information on drug use, extramarital affairs, etc. by FDNY EMS management so beware, and be very, very petrified. To my brother and sister EMT's and paramedics safe tour, God bless and it has been an honor serving with you.

One

Against The Odds

I glanced out of the windshield of the unit as we sat at Forty-second Street and Broadway. The steam rose from the concrete sidewalks as a gentle drizzle soaked the streets. The bus windows were beaded with dancing droplets of water. The FM radio played "You Belong to the City" by Glenn Frey. God, how I loved this job! Having spent three years as an EMT and finally becoming a paramedic in the eighties, I could not ask for more.

EMS, for the most part, ran itself in the streets. Dispatchers *knew* and *listened* to their units. A majority of units would go to the wall backing each other up. The cops might be the Finest, FD the Bravest, but NYC EMS was by and far the Smartest doing over a million calls a year. That was more than any country did! EMS Command was there, but like fleas they were more a nuisance than a threat.

Looking to my right, my partner and friend, Jack Ng, alias Hop Sing, Little Wonton, was fast asleep. It was because of paramedics like Jack, Billy Simon, Miriam Arnold, Burt Meade and other "legends" that I busted my ass to become the best paramedic I could. During my early years in EMS pre-FD hostile takeover, the environment was electrifyingly rich with mentoring for those who wanted to learn from the best. But that was then, this was now.

Jack came to Bellevue Hospital and became my partner on "One Oh Zebra" or, as I answered the radio, "Stress Free, One Oh Zee."

He served as a mechanic in the U.S. Air Force and was kidded about me becoming an Army paratrooper because he was the mechanic of the plane, to the chagrin of our co-workers. He told all who listened that EMS was trying to get him killed because he was Chinese. His partner for years had been Tommy Giorgi, one of the Legends of Harlem. An army veteran, Tommy had what you might call a bad day in Vietnam. First, he was wounded. Then the armored personnel carrier evacuating him was hit and he sustained additional wounds.

Jack had read about "flashbacks" asking "What would you do if I came to work wearing black pajamas and a coolie hat?" I informed him, his wife would find him dead with a 'Screaming Eagle' patch stuffed in his mouth. That ended his quest to be a fashion trendsetter.

When called "Hop Sing," Jack would retort, "Okay, Mr. Cartwright," referring to the well-known sixties TV show, Bonanza. Ethnicity was nothing new in EMS and when used for other than good natured bantering all present recognized that the person hiding behind race, religion or rank was a loser. We dealt with and interacted with America's melting pot of cultures serving and learning from each. On this job you didn't last very long if you were white and couldn't take being called a "cracker" by a Jamaican or "White Nigger" by civilian of color who in his own way was saying thank you. It was part of being part of the EMS family and working the often dark streets of New York City. Most of us acknowledged the uniqueness of others and had fun with it much to the dismay of the purported pencil pushing puritan bosses. We were living the American dream, enjoying life as Comedian Carlos Mencia would say _with feeling_, not being politically correct, afraid of offending anyone. The result was an appreciation of other cultures, and a lot of laughter.

As the music played, he stirred. It was 1:00 a.m. and time to go home. I straightened up in the seat to work the kinks out of my back and the cramps out of my legs. We in

NYC EMS, now the forgotten children of the fire department, lived in these buses for eight to sixteen hours at a stretch. Yet no one had thought to make them comfortable. Thank God for my Chiropractor Dr.Ron Csillag. I reached over and woke Jack.

Damn, the radio just blared. They were calling us. I swear these units are bugged. They always seemed to know when we'd just gotten our food, sat on the bowl, or were about to go home.

Dispatcher: "One Oh Zebra?"

"Stress free One Oh Zee here," I answered. "We're anything, but stress free at the moment."
"Eight David is requesting your assistance. I'm sending you the job via computer. It's a cardiac."
"Ten-Four. Send me the location and have a ten-twelve, presentation of the situation."
"Ten-four."

"Eight David, Central," Lori in the unit responded.

"Give a twelve to Oh Zebra, please."

"We have an eighty-six-year-old male, full blown APE." (Acute pulmonary edema—the left side of the heart is having problems pumping freshly oxygenated blood, so that it backs up. The patient was drowning in his own blood.) Lori spoke into the radio in a stressed, annoyed voice, not like her usual self. I asked for the vital signs. Then she switched into job mode and delivered a great presentation.
She went back to being her calm self and requested an ETA (estimated time of arrival) for our unit.
Dispatcher: "Stress Free, can you give them an ETA?"

I responded, "Tell the unit not to fear. Stress Free One Oh Zee is very near."

As we pulled away from the curb, the lights came on, the siren wailed, and I increased speed. Jack was fully awake now. He rechecked the job on the computer as we careened through the concrete canyons of Manhattan at military speed to save another life.
Singing a little too out loud I caught Jack looking at me.

"What?"

"Who are you singing to?"

"My wife," Melanie had died before our second year together at the age of twenty six.

"Ever think that's why she died to get away from you?"

"Hey, fuck you," I said laughing now really starting to sing out loud.

"Day Oh! Day-a-a oh, one a.m. and we want to go home!

BLS on the scene screaming for a 'rush'

Daylight gone and we want to go home.

They are saying they only want us…" Now Jack joined in.

"Daylight gone and we want to go home!

Day-oh. Day-a-a-oh daylight gone and we want to go home.

We don't care if you're white or you're black.

So long as you have a knife in your back! Hey!

Day-oh. Day-a-a-oh One a.m. and we want to go home.

One body, two body, three body, more

Drug deal went bad so they shot them at the door! Hey!

Day-Oh! Day-a-a-oh, Daylight gone and we want to go home.

We can push lido! We can push dope! We can save your life when there ain't no hope!"

Before the next stanza we were there.

"Stress Free with a pair, Central."

We pulled up to the job location. The rain fell in earnest as I grabbed the drug bag and cardiac monitor. Jack grabbed the oxygen and the Ambulance Call Report (ACR).

I was thinking the patient would need nitroglycerin, an IV, Lasix, morphine, and possible intubation (tube placed down the windpipe to assist patient breathing).

"Come on, Jack. I'm older than you are, can carry more, and still can climb stairs faster!"

And climb the stairs we did. As usual, the elevator in the old building was not running. But the rodents certainly were. We cautiously entered the dim, dank-smelling hallway.

Jack and I both uttered low curses as a rat ran behind two bags of open garbage. The smell of urine made its way from the elevator shaft to our noses.

"Now you know why I call elevators 'vertical urinals,'" I humorously remarked.

Having worked as an elevator repair helper with New York City housing for five years, before leaving to become an EMT and later a paramedic.

We turned right onto a staircase. With one hand I adjusted the drug bag that was digging into my shoulder,

9

while holding the cardiac monitor in the other. Jack adjusted his load, the oxygen bag and ACR (piece of paper). We started climbing the dark stairwell, guided by a dim, dirty bulb on the upper floor.

Passing an open window we were greeted with the smell of rotting garbage from mattresses, rusting cans, and newspapers. The unwanted refuse dumped from various apartment windows into the courtyard, having been neglected by the superintendent, fire inspectors, and the sanitation department. Not even the fresh summer rain could drown the stench.

Passing the third floor I heard a dog, a very big dog, howling behind a chained door. There was no doorknob, just a heavy chain threaded through a hole in the wall, where the doorknob should have been. The pit bull went ballistic, howling and scratching to get at us. I hoped the inside was secured with a heavy padlock. I heard a drunk-sounding male yell at the dog in slurred Spanish, as a TV blared a Spanish soap program.

Continuing to make our way up the stairwell, we stepped over two junkies in our path. As we hugged the inside wall, a thin, black male grabbed two glowing pipes, so we would not step on them. A female was servicing him. Her filthy jeans and soiled, yellow panties were pulled down to her knees. She was naked to the waist. Her back and arms showed multiple, inflamed sores and needle tracks. Kneeling on the steps below the male, she looked worse than a Mike Tyson date. From the rear, she reminded me of the water buffaloes I had seen in the rice paddies of Vietnam. No disrespect meant to the buffaloes.

"Thank you," I said as we climbed the steps where the pipes had been. Every little bit of public cooperation helps on this job.

The black male gave a half-stoned smile, jaundiced eyes showing a lackluster emptiness. He waved the glowing pipes. The crack in the pipe bowls glowed red and smoke drifted in a lazy stream. The girl attempted to look up at us, but he pushed her head back down with a slap. Opening her mouth, exposing one gold tooth among gaps and thrush she took his dark, shriveled penis, in hand. The man smacked her head again as she attempted one last look at us. With her drooling mouth and bloodshot eyes, she went back to work.

We finally got to the fifth floor, which was actually the sixth floor. We cursed the idiot who designed the building so the first floor was marked the main floor and apartment 5A was on the sixth floor. By now both of us were huffing and puffing.

Naked light bulbs cast the cold, gloomy light. Chipped paint littered the floors and bare wires hung from the ceiling. We looked for 5A, but most of the doors in the hallway were not even numbered. The doors were labeled using magic markers and covered with stickers, such as "Jesus Saves," "Our Lady of Guadeloupe," "Free Puerto Rico." Others had graffiti with graphic explanations of who did what, where, and to whom. Some boasted of the toughest gang and the names of girls to provide a good time, with telephone numbers and the costs.

"Candy Love" seemed to be the girl who got around as her name appeared on the walls on several floors. Someone spray painted "The Duke is Dead, RIP" in red paint. The response was spray painted in blue, "So is Buckwheat."

Everyone seemed to love mothers, since "Your Mother" appeared everywhere. This must be a real happening place on Mother's Day, I chuckled.

We spotted the open door at the extreme end of the hall. In EMS Land one can always count on the last call being a walkup, at the end of a long hall, the patient being a "quarter-pounder with cheese" (morbidly overweight), and the job being real—the patient actually needs paramedics. Stepping on two wrapped syringes and a spent condom, I walked to the door. It was comforting to know some people were using clean needles and condoms. Clean sex and clean needles make for a happy junkie high.

This door was decorated with a dried corn husk, a rubber snake, and more condoms. It was blocked open with the EMTs' Heart Start Defibrillator, or, as we all call it, the 'Door Stopper'.

I heard a commotion but couldn't make out the voices. Jack and I stood on either side of the door, in case shots were fired. I yelled for the crew to answer us. We heard EMT Jim Conners, "The Lip," yell to hurry up. Jimmy and I were EMT partners years ago in Spanish Harlem.

He got his nickname because "Lip" was tattooed on the inside of his lower lip. Being the biggest, I went through the door first entering the dark living room and following a harsh light from a room at the extreme end of the hall. Passing the kitchen, I noticed it was loaded with old newspapers and dishes were piled high in the sink. A cat was perched on the counter, licking water from a dish in the sink as roaches scurried about.

We entered a well-lit bedroom. Jim was behind a tall, Morbidly overweight, Caucasian male, sixty years old, wearing only an old torn dingy yellow T-shirt stained with blood. The light reflected off the old man's sweat-soaked body. He was sitting tripod in a chair pushing and twisting his body to get free from the BVM (bag valve mask) Jim was holding over his nose and mouth. With all his strength, the old man was fighting to rip off the mask while screaming that he couldn't breathe. Jim fought with all his might to keep a tight fit over the old man's nose and mouth attempting to use positive pressure to breathe for the man who was drowning in his own fluid. We could hear the wet gurgles coming from him as he tried harder to scream.

Relaxing a moment after the climb and doing a quick 10 second survey, Jim greeted us with full respect, "'Bout time you prima donna medics got here!" In this split second, the old man pushed the mask out of Jim's hands as it went flying to the floor. The patient lunged forward from the chair, making a death knell sound, eyes grotesquely bulged with horror as copious amounts of pink and red fluid violently erupted from his nose and mouth. He was drowning, medically known as APE (Acute Pulmonary Edema).

Reaching from behind the worn chair, Jim managed to grab the old man's T-shirt, yanking him forcefully into the chair in an upright position. He yelled for Lori, his partner to pass him the BVM from the floor and attach it back to the oxygen bottle.

Lori stood frozen by the bedside table. Her sunny face was blank, beautiful hair hung in disarray, uniform soaked in sweat. Small, graceful hands trembled in the dark blue protective gloves.

Yelling again, no reaction, the eyes told the story wide with paralyzing fear, like a deer caught in the headlights of a speeding car. I've seen this look before in combat and knew Jim's screams would not reach her. She was overwhelmed and lost. In combat if a soldier wasted time on such a person, it usually cost him his life. So without a word, I passed the BVM to Jim and hooked it to the hissing oxygen tank.

As Jim held the mask firmly, sealing it as best he could on the blood and sputum-soaked face, the old man stopped fighting. Jim firmly compressed the bag, trying to get oxygen into the lungs and push the fluid back. The red-tinged fluid continued to escape from around the mask.

The old man was getting weaker, his respirations slowing. He was dying right in front of us. So began the choreographed ballet EMS crews perform day and night, under all conditions, against all odds, to save a life.

I quickly opened the drug bag and passed the intubation set to my left. Jack grabbed it like a pro running back for the New York Jets, proceeding to Jim's left, setting up to intubate the man. To intubate, we place a plastic tube down the trachea. The neck houses the trachea and the esophagus. The trachea runs from the mouth to the lungs, carrying oxygen in and waste out during breathing. Behind the trachea, is the esophagus, which goes from the mouth to stomach. During intubation, the tube seals off the stomach, allowing us to deliver oxygen into the lungs and remove wasteful gases. Also, it provides a route for some medication.

I set up to get an IV into the man to deliver life-saving drugs. With street-learned precision that would put the New York Ballet to shame, Jim moved to his left dropping the BVM to his side as Jack started to place the tube down the man's throat. The man made a weak, futile attempt to swivel his head away. Jim held it in place as Jack told the man that without this tube to help him breathe, he would die.

I saw the eyes of the old man as I positioned to put the IV in his soaked, slippery, dirty arm. His eyes, the true indicator of the soul, reflected a grim, haunting acceptance and confusion, yet not the 'faraway' look we all know. When a patient has the faraway look, an eerie, diabolical emptiness devoid of life is seen, and you know the dance of life is over. At that moment the soul leaves the body, and no matter what we do, it is not coming back. Usually right before that as the patient is circling the drain I hear 'Knock, knock, knocking on Heavens Door' playing in my head.

We were still in the fight with a viable patient. The old man gagged, as Jack stood on his toes behind the chair, trying to get a better view inside his blood-bubbling mouth. There would be no time to suction him prior to the tube. Jack was sweating, as Jim tilted the chair back expertly applying hand pressure on the man's throat to help Jack visualize the trachea. Just as Jim tilted the chair, I was going into the only vein I saw in his arm and blew it! I hated days like this.

Jim realized what happened, and I heard a muttered curse and apology as he wiped his sweat-soaked face on his shirtsleeve. No time to look up. The priority was the tube, so we could breathe for the old man. As we all know, breathing is a good thing.

Although we could deliver medicine down the tube, it is not the best route. I searched again for a vein, uttering a silent prayer to my Spirit Guides. I didn't see a vein in his neck, scalp, or arms, but I found a great one in his filthy foot. "Thanks," I muttered hearing Jack ask Jim to hold the tube while he checked for lung sounds, to ensure the tube was in place. It was. I was having a problem securing the IV line because the man's skin was so wet. As I knelt on his foot so he couldn't move it and lose the IV, I grabbed a four-by-four bandage and opened it with my teeth. Next, I reached for the alcohol, the patient's alcohol, Jack Daniels. Dousing the four-by-four, then rubbing it over the foot. The alcohol dried up the sweat and I could now apply several layers of tape to hold the line in place. Jack completed intubating the patient and took a fast blood pressure.

He remarked about my drinking habits on the job while attempting to hook up the cardiac monitor. Needless to say the EKG pasties would not stick, so he asked for the bottle of alcohol. Jim had the BVM attached to the end of the intubation tube and now matched the patient's attempts at breathing. He helped him draw easier, fuller breaths.

"I'm gonna contact CCU (Civilian Complaint Unit), to report you two prima-donna White Patches using liquor on the job. The patient's liquor! What do you think, you're bucket fairies?" Jim uttered. ("Bucket fairies" was one of many terms used to refer to firemen.). He has such a way with words.

As Jack called out the vital signs and headed toward the phone to call telemetry for clearance on morphine, I placed a nitroglycerin pill under the patient's tongue. This would help lower his blood pressure on the right side of the heart. Sending less blood into the right side meant less blood on the left and, consequently, less to back up into his lungs. A drier surface in the lungs meant better oxygen and waste exchange.

Next, to help the heart get rid of excess fluid, I gave him eighty milligrams of furosimide (Lasix) through the IV. It usually takes twenty minutes for the patient to rid his body of excess fluid, to urinate. But medicine is an art, not a science.

Pushing the Lasix through his foot vein, I felt and smelled the fruit of my labor. The patient pissed on me. In my career, I had only two patients void as soon as I gave this drug. But none had ever given me a golden shower. I jumped up, grabbed a shirt off the bed, and threw it onto his genital area to absorb the foul, pungent, golden spray.

Jim looked at me as I cursed. Laughing so much, he was out of sync with the patient's breathing. As the patient gagged to breathe, it appeared he too was laughing at the situation. I looked at both, yelling to Jim, "Fuck both of you, and watch his breathing, "Piss Patch." (Piss Patch is what I lovingly call the EMTs at Bellevue.) Jack returned remarking, "We're clear on the morphine up to eight milligrams at increments of two after an initial four." Looking at me, noticing that my sleeve was soaked, he commented, "You really need to shower more often."

"Fuck you. Just draw up the morphine, Hop Sing." This got a laugh from everyone.

The morphine helped to calm the patient and decreased the heart load. We completed another set of vital signs, another twelve-lead EKG, then started to package him and our equipment.

Lori had become responsive enough to open the folding chair, in which we placed the patient. We would carry this intubated patient in the chair, using gravity to assist us in drawing fluid to the lower parts of his lungs.

As we were packaging the patient, a voice called out and two cops walked in. They were late as usual, but we were glad to see them. They offered to carry the equipment. When we reached the hallway, I took the bottom of the chair, with one officer behind me guiding my steps. Jim took the top of the chair, with the IV bag attached to his shirt. Jack, being smaller, stood sideways, assisting the patient's breathing by squeezing the BVM with the oxygen bottle on the patient's lap. Lori walked in silence, carrying equipment. The other officer secured the door to the apartment and carried the rest of the equipment.

Flight after dangerous flight we went down, each of us watching the other and the patient. I swore out loud that if the patient started to urinate again, I was going to drop him. Everyone laughed.

Turn after tight turn, the pain in my back was matched by the exertion of the others, as shown by the expressions on their faces.

"Yeah, I can see myself doing this till I'm sixty-two," Jim said.

"What's the matter, son, can't handle it?" I volleyed.

"Keep it up and I'll let Jack carry the chair," he threatened. Ah, the love.

On the ground floor we wheeled, pulled, and dragged the chair to the lobby entrance. Back spasms tore through my body as I straightened up.

Going outside into the cool, rain-soaked night I opened the back of the bus (ambulance) and get a blanket to cover the old man. I took a deep, lung-filling breath, looked out into the dark, rainy night and whispered a heartfelt "Thank you."

The cold water soaking me felt like a blessed embrace. My body ached, yet it felt good to be alive and team up with these special people.

Outside, we worked with precision in silence. In the back of the bus, we redid vital signs and an EKG. Both had improved. The patient's color and lung sounds were much better. I tied his hands to the stretcher in case he started to get agitated and attempted to pull out the intubation tube. Changing the portable oxygen bottle, I explained to the patient that everything would be all right and if he understood to raise his left index finger.

The finger came up. Jim continued to assist the patient's breathing.

Jack gave him another two milligrams of morphine. Both he and Jim would remain in the back, while I drove our unit and Lori drove them to Bellevue Hospital.

Although we were on the West Side of Manhattan and there was St. Vincent's, St. Claire's, and Roosevelt Hospitals, we knew Bellevue Hospital on First Avenue and

East Twenty eighth Street was the best for the patient. Bellevue is a city hospital where my wife died of an aneurysm at the age of twenty-seven. I came to work at Bellevue years later and stayed because of the medical staff.

Lori was already up front in the driver's seat, isolating herself from us and awaiting the signal to move. The cops standing under the protective awning called for an ACR number. I called it out to them. Jack sat on the crew bench, Jim sat behind the patient, still assisting him to breathe. The patient was much more comfortable now. Standing in the soft rain, I asked if Jack had everything.

"Yeah, I'm fine."

Looking at the patient his eyes no longer terror filled and the confusion was gone. I closed the door and walked to my bus. I was in the lead as we started across town. People were still walking on the Manhattan streets, but there were fewer of them now and less traffic. The neon lights reflected the rain-soaked streets of the greatest city in the world.

As we pulled onto the grounds of Bellevue Hospital, the East River was to my left. The fog slowly rolled in, but I could see the soft blue lights of the emergency room sign. It guided us to the ambulance bay, which was encased in a yellow glow from the overhead lighting. Lori backed into the ambulance bay, as I parked some distance away, against the fence hitting the signal on the computer and exiting the bus. I was struck by the sweet smell of salt water in the air, as the rain subsided. Looking to my right wild, yellow roses silently graced the fence next to the emergency room. Often I'd walk over and take a whiff, but not now.

Lori had the back door of the bus open. I asked how the patient was doing and Jack said, "Fine." Two crew members came out to give us a hand with the lift. As we pulled him out, I grabbed the left side of the stretcher and EMTs Karl Dykman and Ashley Alejo, two of my favorite Piss Patches at Bellevue, grabbed the other side. Jim assisted the patient's breathing while Jack got the release at the end of the stretcher.

As we pulled him out I remarked, "Sure two of you young warriors on one side and me, the ancient one, left alone on this side."

Jack remarked, "Well, if you wouldn't piss on yourself..."

The EMTs looked and Jim said, "Yeah, the patient pissed on Stress Free over there."

I just laughed uttering, "Let's get him inside before he dies of pneumonia."

Once inside, the smell of the Jack Daniels rubdown preceded us. A new triage nurse remarked, "Oh, another drunk? We've had our fill . . ." then stopped mid-sentence when she saw he was tubed.

Drs. Bob Hoffman and Dave Jacobs, two of Bellevue's best, came out and asked what we had. Jack did a five-second presentation, as both doctors began to pull the stretcher into the emergency room area. Flustered, the nurse walked behind the patient, Jack, Jim, Karl, Ashley, and the doctors, complaining she had not yet done the triage.

I walked back outside onto the ramp taking a deep breath, Lori walked by, stopped, looked at me, and then proceeded to open the back door of her vehicle. Without a word, I retrieved the drug bag and monitor and walked to my vehicle. After the re-stock the rain stopped. I walked over, asked permission of the roses, before taking a whiff. Thanking them as I walked back and stood in front of our bus, waiting for Jack to finish his paperwork. The gentle perfume of the roses, mixed with the saltwater mist, created a heavenly elixir placing me at peace.

Lori sat stoically in her unit. In one terrifying moment becoming lost, recognizing her mortality in this patient; *becoming* this patient and could only watch as death approached. Her fairy-tale-oriented ideas of glory, saving the patient, being the heroine, were eternally smashed. In that split second she couldn't scream, cry, or even save herself, the morphosis had happened. In one crushing moment her mortality stood real, as the bestial whisper of death approached with a stark chill.

She could leave the job or compound the lie by completing a paramedic program and getting the coveted "White Patch." Two things were guaranteed. First, she would never have the heart to be a real street paramedic, like the legendary Miriam Arnold, William Simons, and others.

Lori might graduate and with no time on the streets, go into Inspectional Services, or become a chief's aide with the help of her looks and emotional manipulations.

Perhaps, she might even come back to Bellevue to work a shift of overtime when I'm off, so she wouldn't have to face me. Perhaps one day she would indeed become an officer or even chief. Any of us with time on the job had seen certain females 'work' their way up from 'below,' on their knees, while other females like Miriam, and Lt. Kate Vinkus quietly did their jobs professionally and with honor. But the lie would always haunt her. As she rose in rank, she would look with both outward disdain and silent wonder at the real heroes and heroines of this job. Deep in the silence of her soul, she would know that every one of these street EMTs and paramedics had faced the same stark terror, recognition of their own mortality and death, but chose to fight on.

Secondly, and more sadly, EMS Command would never provide meaningful aid to assist people like Lori. Years later the FD would make a superficial attempt at "screening" out those who the pencil-pushing psychologist pundits "judged" unfit. The reality was some along the way would be lost to suicide, drugs or alcohol. But the majority of street personnel would continue against the odds. All likes and dislikes aside, these New York City street EMTs and paramedics are silent saints in a very noble profession.

Jack and I drove back to the garage at Battalion Eight, the Kipps Bay Station. Located on the Bellevue Hospital grounds, it's reportedly the oldest municipal ambulance garage in the United States. Jack asked how I was doing. He realized what had just transpired with Lori and realized I liked her.

He also knew this was the twenty-fifth anniversary of my wife's death. Melanie, my best friend and soul mate, died before our second year of marriage in 1975.

Jack said if it were him, he'd spend the night with a girl, not here on the streets. His voice drifted off, as I thanked him for a good night and went into the office to sign the narcotics and radio in.

After cleaning up, Lieutenant Ralph Ortiz gave me a lift to Grand Central Station at Forty-second Street and Lexington Avenue. Approaching the escalators, I walked past the homeless lying on the floor under one of the most marvelous cathedral ceilings ever created. I proceeded down past more homeless on benches by the token booth and onto the number seven train. Finding an empty car I sat alone watching the rain water streak across the glass and wondered how much this job had changed and how it had changed me.

Two
EMS
Where ... Every Minute Sucks

When I first joined EMS in 1983, we were *not* part of FDNY, but rather Health and Hospitals Corp. Within this environment one could move on to become a respiratory tech, nurse, or paramedic. Either way, the worker, hospitals, city and patient gained by keeping experienced workers. I was content for a brief period of time to be an EMT at King's County Hospital in the heart of Brooklyn.

In those days we were called "The Tombstones" because of the patch's shape. As I watched and learned from the likes of Billy, Sandy and Miriam, I couldn't help but be caught up in wanting to know more so I could do more for the patient. Learning was contagious around these three, because they encouraged me. They always found time to answer questions, which instilled confidence.

I had left the County to work at Station Fifteen at Metropolitan Hospital on Ninety-seventh Street and First Avenue in Manhattan.

I was totally captivated by the electric environment of the Spanish culture. The girls were stunning in richly colored dresses, with pouting, sensuous lips below sparkling, almond eyes. Big, gold hoop earrings swayed to the rhythm of life offsetting black, shoulder-length hair. The rhythm was accented by a music that demanded attention. The Latino beat permeated the neighborhood day and night, reflecting both the hope and vitality of this working-class neighborhood. The music and beauty of the girls was second only to the hospitality and humor of the Spanish culture.

At Station Fifteen, Metropolitan Hospital, I met Lieutenant Manny Barrios. Manny was a real Latin lover, in his mind. His life typified Hispanic flare and humor. He became a good friend to the troops under him often going out of his way when our alcoholic captain attempted to fry the troops. His mode of operation (MO) would be to talk to us about his boat one minute, knifing us in the back the next. This loser retired as a captain. At his retirement party, the chief and others told him he should stay,

"There's a place for you with us chiefs." Yeah, the bullshit really flowed. But in those days the troops were basically isolated from the whims and bad judgment calls of the EMS brass by people like Manny. For the most part, we street people only had contact with immediate supervision during roll calls or signing out radios. The chiefs remained in their isolated little kingdoms.

Backstabbing wasn't anything new, but in the Barrio, certain captains went at it with zest. It was a trademark.

One in communications went out drinking with the dispatchers and then told the floor lieutenant to write them up for this or that. He had the makings the chiefs were looking for, so he was later promoted.

In October 1986, the street crews had had enough of the nonsense dished out by EMS Chief Robert Becker and the City concerning our contract. We all agreed we deserved better pay, pensions, and benefits but we were too professional to take it out on the public, whom we willingly served. Instead decided to report for duty and serve the public, but we would not wear the EMS uniform. It was a citywide deal.

On the designated night, I reported in, refusing to go out to the unit in uniform. ISU (Inspectional Service Unit) was waiting so they could make their threats and write us up. They silently stood around, not talking to anyone in the garage, like a pack of rabid wildly deranged wolves waiting to pounce. With each refusal their frenzy of delight grew at writing us violations.

The first one to receive his violation was Lieutenant Steve Lawrence. He was the boss behind the desk. Never known for his "gentle mannerisms," Steve just about threw the off-coming tour out the door. We learned later that the darlings of ISU, Becker's Gestapo, were trying to get Steve to mandate the tour or have them sent home with charges.

The reason? The city would be saved from embarrassment by those "EMS people." EMS administration, for their part, claimed that they were only concerned for our safety. It was all a smokescreen to hide the gods' uneasiness with these malcontents who were demanding better pay, working conditions and equipment for the patients.

As for the troops, I proudly reported in, the first on our tour to receive a violation. I signed for it, went out, and started checking the unit.

While I was checking out the vehicle, the passenger side opened and a uniformed EMT introduced himself as Jim Conners.

"I'll be working with you tonight. I'm new."

"Not dressed like that, you won't be working with me," I said in my gentle, loving manner. Jim got out, went to the garage, and changed. This took a lot of courage. EMS later fired these new people for their act of solidarity. But Jim held in there and became a great EMT and friend.

We got the reaction we wanted from both the public and the New York City administration, led by the all-knowing pompous Mayor Ed Koch.

The last time the city was annoyed by those "EMS people" was back in the early part of 1970. The crews at the Harlem Hospital garage refused to go out. The EMT corps was established between 1963 and 1965. Five years later, they were still without the most basic of equipment they needed to serve the public. Was there discrimination?

You bet. In those days, EMTs were predominantly black. Today we still are staffed with a majority of minorities. But now there is a very rich diversity within our ranks.

The African-Americans of EMS Harlem led the way for our action almost eighteen years later as the noble fight between healers and pundits/administrators continued.

As you'll read later toward the end of my career with NYC the political faces change but this lack of appropriate cutting edge technology to save your life used in other agencies across the nation, some used by voluntary hospital paramedic units still has not found itself into the largest EMS system in the world. The other hidden dirty secret was the money. Not our paycheck but how much money the city charged for our treating you. Years later Local 2507 would pit us against the "voluntary hospitals (St. Claire's, NY Cornell, etc.) and for profit ambulance service (ie MetroCare)" never acknowledging that there never was, nor is a 'free' non charging NYC EMS. It's interesting since when the firefighters put out a fire in your house you don't receive a bill. When the police breakup a family fight, you don't get a bill. But when EMS responds, the third part of the Trinity of Emergency Service, you and the rest of us tax payers _are_ charged. Has anyone read the original mandate for EMS? So once again it is not about patient care, it is about the money. Keep an eye on this concept as you learn how the whole system was perverted.

During these years I was flying medical evacuation missions as a flight medic with the Air Force Reserves. One EMT chief went out of his way to bust my shoes concerning the flying missions. He demanded to know where I was going and when. It crossed the line with me. I gave notification a month in advance of my flight it would help with EMS staffing. But as with all attempts with these inept wonders that ran EMS, it wasn't good enough. Or in the infamous words of my friend paramedic Harvey Feintuch, "No good deed will go unpunished."

By law, I only needed to tell the EMS station I was leaving the night before, and upon returning, hand in orders when I was on active duty. Under *no circumstances* did they have the right, or security clearance, to know where I was flying on worldwide missions.

One night, the chief was in the office with an ISU officer at his side. He made wise-ass remarks about my flights. Doubting he ever served in *our* armed forces, because he would have never made such disparaging remarks about those who served. "Excuse me, Chief. Do you like running off at the mouth concerning my military activities?"

The ISU officer perked up, figuring he had me on a solid case of insubordination. The chief developed diarrhea of the mouth. I stood there and listened until I'd had enough. He was in mid-sentence, as I reached in my pocket, removed the miniature tape recorder, and held it in front of his silent, wide-open mouth. To say he and his buddy were in shock was an understatement.

Turning off the tape recorder starting to walk outside; "You really should think before you make asshole statements."

While outside, talking to a crew the chief came storming past, I remarked to a crew, "And this item should be carried whenever talking to chiefs." Once in his car he couldn't move, my personal car was blocking his. Rolling down the window he meekly asked whose car it was? I told him it was mine and would be there in a moment... *after I was done*. As he sat and burned, I said my goodnights to the crew, walked over, and tapped on his window. He lowered it, "Good night, Chief." Then I got into my car.

They never learn. Several days later, I was ordered to report to Location One, 'Puzzle Palace', to see "Judge Woppner" concerning my military activity. Judge Woppner, as we called Bill Leask, a reported retired NYPD ESU police officer that meted punishments to those who went afoul. Funny thing, no one ever accounted for the money from these fines. Having had enough, I called my wing commander at McGuire Air Force Base who contacted another friend at the Pentagon. Once the friend heard what was requested, he agreed it constituted harassment and was a serious security breach.

On the morning I was to report to Judge Woppner, Lt. Barrios told me, "Go back to your unit, Poppy."

"Why, what's up?"

"I don't know nor care to know who *you know*. But a phone call went into Chief Becker at Maspeth. The result—hands off."

As usual, these clowns never learn.

Later, when my buddy the Chief was out on a line-of-duty injury (LODI), he was set up by "his buddies" and caught making a pizza delivery. He was not as secure as he thought with the other gods who didn't like his mouth. It seemed he wasn't playing nice with them and was busted to lieutenant, thus the nickname, 'Pizza Man'.

I gave him a lot of credit for coming back to work, unlike Chief Becker whose day was coming. This hapless chief, then lieutenant, had the misfortune of having his wife show up at the apartment of a busty EMT while he was there. The wife demanded to know why she was 'doing' her husband. The lieutenant was moved to another borough.

The EMT divorced and left the service leaving fond memories, well for some anyway.

Working the streets, I learned a lot from great partners and even those who weren't that great. It was a cold and rainy day in Spanish Harlem. The sky was overcast with a low ceiling of rain clouds. For the most part, the streets were abandoned. Some junkies, alcoholics, and street people gathered around trash cans, where the burning wood and paper which served as a heater. The dreary weather matched the depressed feelings on the street.

We received a call to respond to the Twenty-third Police Precinct located at One Hundred Second Street in Spanish Harlem for a "rape." My partner, Vinny Hanlon, and I arrived at the precinct being ushered to the side by a female police officer, who held something in a sheet over the heater. A male officer was talking to her and trying to ensure the bundle would not get too hot. Another female saw us,

"Thank God you guys are here."

"What's up?" I asked.

She opened the bundle to show us a six-month-old baby. Her name; Desiree.

"She's been sexually abused," the male officer uttered before starting to scream, "I'll kill those sons of bitches! How could this happen?"

The officer who brought her in started crying and a male officer hugged him. A female officer put her arms around both of them and directed them away.

"Let me see her," I said, wanting to ensure she had no immediate life-threatening injury.

I found a table and started to examine the baby. The baby's rectum was bruised and indeed there were scratches and bruises on her body. She had been violated rectally.

The mother and the live-in boyfriend were junkies. The mother was selling the baby for drugs. The boyfriend got scared so he decided to bring in this bundle of love walking into the precinct holding the naked, wet baby.

I took off my green EMS coat and spread it on the table, placing precious Desiree within. To this day I can still see her beautiful, long, black eyelashes. Vinny opened the bus and I got in with an officer. On the way, I wet my finger and baptized Desiree, never wanting to let her go. And after all these years I now *know* I never did let her go since she is still in my heart.

Another great partner was Octavio Olivieri, known as "Al" by his friends. He was a former paramedic who, for whatever reasons, gave up the patch. One night Al and I were working the 11:00 p.m. to 7:00 a.m. shift.

At 5:00 a.m., the dispatcher called, "One Four Boy? Four Bad Boys?"

I answered, "Bad Boys here. How can we help you?"

"Bad Boys, your modat is driving us crazy. Please turn it off." The modat was our mobile radio in the unit.

"Okay, turning it off," I responded and looked at Al. We both smiled. It was a beautiful Sunday morning as we drove to a Spanish eatery. We ambled inside and ordered, admiring and joking with the waitress, leisurely eating breakfast. We bought newspapers and read them drinking more great Spanish coffee. By the time we were finished, the sun was up and it was about a quarter to quitting time. We drove back to the garage at Metropolitan Hospital very relaxed.

Walking into the office to sign out and were greeted by an agitated Lieutenant Barrios.

"Where the hell have you guys been?" he asked.

Al responded, "Having breakfast, reading the papers, why?"

"Why didn't you guys answer the damn radio?"

"Because they told us to turn it off," I responded.

Now Manny, normally a cool lieutenant, looked bewildered.

"I know that. But why didn't you turn it back on?" he demanded.

"Because no one said to turn it on, only off," I said with a smile, totally flustering him.

"The tour commander wants you to call." I looked at my watch and it was a minute after seven.

"Al, you want the overtime to call?"

"No, I'm going home to enjoy the rest of the day."

"Yeah, me too. Tell the tour commander we'd like to talk to him, but that would require us getting overtime we don't want. Good night, Manny." Both of us walked. Manny received more practice on being a saint.

One of the great pleasures of working out of Metropolitan in Spanish Harlem was the officers in the Twenty-fourth Precinct. There were several whom we really enjoyed.

One night, Jim and I had pulled over a "livery" cab going the wrong way on Amsterdam Avenue. It had almost hit some kids crossing the street. As the kids ran into the street looking in the direction of the oncoming traffic, the driver came from the other direction. Fast thinking, I hit the siren to get the kids' attention and threw on the lights to wake up the driver. Then cut the driver off with the bus.

"Give me your license, registration, and green card," I demanded of the driver.

The confused driver handed it over I passed them to Jim (The Lip) who walked back to the bus.

"Do you realize you almost hit those kids driving the wrong way?" I asked.

The driver came up with excuses as locals stopped, cursed at the driver and thanked us for the fast work. As I lectured the driver, Jim did an 'immigration check' on the modat. He placed the documents into a slot on the computer console.

The driver figured it was the real deal. As we awaited the return of the 'signal,' a sergeant from the Twenty-fourth Precinct pulled up. Without getting out, he asked, "Doing immigration checks?"

"Yeah, Sarge."

"Well, if you get a collar, let us know, and we'll transport."

With a wave, the sergeant was gone and the driver was sweating a bit more. Jim returned the documents and admonished the guy.

One night, we were out and about when I noticed in my mirror a car traveling wildly up Amsterdam Avenue. Both of us watched as it careened through traffic. A white male was at the wheel and a black male was in the passenger seat. So far it had blown two red lights as it traveled north. We spotted a Twenty-fourth Precinct car. Pulling up, we gave the description of the recklessly driven vehicle. I was sitting higher up than the police car and the officer asked, "Do you see them?"

"Yeah, I have a visual."

"Okay, we'll follow you," we were told.

The unit lurched forward, lights and sirens going, and the pursuit was on. The unsuspecting car continued north. Once parallel to the car on Amsterdam and Ninety-fifth Street, I yelled at the passenger, "Pull the vehicle over, now."

"Fuck you, white boy," was the reply.

"Oh yeah, watch this, Stymie."

I cut into the vehicle, ripping part of the car's molding off. A four-foot section of molding was stuck in our rear wheel-well at the same moment we cut the vehicle off, and the sector threw their lights on.

"Thanks, EMS. We'll take it from here," the cops said. The males were charged with grand theft auto. Public education and safety is part of our job.

It was a dark, dismal, foggy night as Vinny and I were out and about. Suddenly we heard a Twenty-fourth Precinct sector put out a call for a backup. It didn't seem urgent, but since Vinny and I weren't too busy, we decided to ride over.

Pulling up to the location shutting down another sector pulled behind us. A woman screamed above us, her voice vibrating through the cold damp fog as she appeared to lunge out of the fourth-floor window. The same moment we saw a cop frantically grab trying to pull the deranged woman in. Before we could get to the entrance of the building, the officer was pulled halfway out the window refusing to release her as his partner now visible fought desperately to pull both back from the brink of death.

I made a mad dash into the lobby and started running up the stairs, Vinny behind, calling over my shoulder which apartment. The answer was passed up from the two cops lagging behind Vinny.

On the floor I located the apartment. Banging loudly on the door, I heard everyone pile onto the landing behind me. The door opened and directly in front of me stood a guy who looked like Alfred E. Newman. He wore a Perry Como sweater with putrid red sneakers holding a Mag light. Behind him stood a man and a woman and to the left was a rug dividing the kitchen from the living room. Behind the curtain we could hear the fighting as the two officers yelled out for help.

Stepping forward, this patsy attempted to shove me with the mag light, so I launched him through the curtain into the next room. Ricocheting off the wall he came at me again.

The cops were wrestling on the floor with an EDP (Every Day Person) and the Perry Como guy was coming at me. I grabbed him, bounced him over the couch and into the wall again. Reaching to help with the EDP Vinny yelled, "Here he comes again!"

The guy came at me a third time! This was getting annoying. Grabbing him by his scrawny throat, I lifted him up, cocked my arm back, fist poised, ready to knock him out. Vinny now screamed, "Hit him. Hit him, Jim!"

The guy was literally off the floor and about to receive the mother of all knockout punches when I heard Officer Hunt yell, "Jim, he's a cop!"

I now forcefully bounced him against the wall again just or good measure. With the fight out of him as well as a flash of sanity entering his pus filled brain, he remained a wallflower as we assisted the cops cuffing the violently thrashing, cursing, biting EDP.

When the Perry Como guy regained composure, he asked, "Are you EMS?"

"No, I'm the fuckin' sanitation man."

"Yeah, they're EMS," said Officer Hunt as he slowly got up.

"Well, put that person in a straitjacket now," the idiot ordered.

"Are you sure this asshole is a cop? Straightjacket?" I asked, looking at the cops.

"Well, I still haven't seen any identification," one of the cops remarked, receiving a death stare from the idiot.

"Neither have I," chimed in my cheerleader, Vinny.

The clown produced not a shield, but plastic identification. It turned out that I had bounced around a police duty captain. He was the captain for the Central Park Precinct. Yeah, he knew about crime. Catching squirrels jaywalking is a bitch. Counting the nuts in their position was intimidating and terrifying police work since he didn't possess any himself.

"Take this person away!" he demanded, looking at me, still trying to gain control.

"Fuck you, asshole. We are not assigned this job, so you call for a bus." I said over my shoulder, following Vinny toward the door.

"Please, guys, for us?"

How could we turn down these cops who were being trailed by the duty captain, risking their lives trying to save another, without the help of this clown. Vinny and I looked at each other.

"Okay," we said in unison.

Vinny got the chair. We loaded the patient onto the chair then all piled into the elevator. It was silent. The police captain looked at me, "You know, I have a gun."

I looked down into his eyes and responded in a low, calm voice. "If you had pulled your gun on me, I would have shoved it up your ass and blown out your brains."

There was a chuckle from one of the cops. The elevator grew warm.

The captain's temperature was going even higher. He looked first at the officer who chuckled, then at me.

"I should have you arrested right now," he said in his most recent authoritarian voice.

"If you put the cuffs on me I will own you, your wife, and your firstborn female child. Both females will be working for me on Forty-second Street. If you are that stupid, please do it."

He stood frozen. The elevator door opened and the cool moist night air rushed in.

Later at Saint Luke's, I heard him say to one of the cops, "I'm really hurt. I want to be seen." I turned, "Want me to do the paperwork, captain?"

A deadly, cold stare met me as I smiled, walking inside.

Good news travels fast in all circles. A little while later, a cop pulled up from the Central Park Precinct. The officer came over to me.

"Are you the guy who punched out my captain?"

"Yeah," I answered, figuring he might want to make an issue out of it.

"Well, why didn't you throw his ass out the window?" he asked with a smile.

Several days later while in the Twenty-third Precinct a few cops said, "Oh, you're the guy."

"Yes, he is," said my cheerleader, Vinny.

"Listen, we have collected some money. Could you do our captain?"

We all laughed. Months later I learned the captain I'd bounced around went to the Twenty-fourth Precinct that night, complaining about, "Getting an injury from a beating by some EMS guy."

It never went further because the cops told their CO (Commanding Officer of the 24 Pct.) what occurred. If push came to shove the cops, along with their CO, would put Vinny and me in for an award.

The captain was later sent to the FBI (Famous But Inept) Academy for classes. I sure hope the G-men taught him what they are most noted for. No, not solving cases, but identifying themselves!

There was a Dunkin' Donut shop on Ninety-sixth Street and Broadway a few steps from Club Broadway. We picked up coffee and donuts or Dominican girls when the club was open. Also we competed with the local sector from the Twenty-fourth Precinct. They tried to beat us into the corner location to check out the girls. One night, we pulled up and two of New York's Finest were there.

"Pardon us, officers, but you are in a designated EMS 14 Boy parking zone," Nelson, my partner said politely.

"Too bad, this is NYPD turf, pal," chuckled the officer his partner talking to a very young, and sensual Dominican young lady.

"Oh really? Well, 'Kind and Informed Defender of the Peace,' there seems to be a gap in your knowledge." I said, raising my portable radio. "But to clarify this matter we shall request your sergeant to the scene."

"Okay. Okay. You dirt bags have it," he said with a huff.

"Dirt bags, you say? No problem."

They pulled out and we pulled in, realizing we would get it later.

Practical jokes flowed both ways. One night, an EMS unit, guess whose, was chased with lights and sirens going from the Twentieth Precinct into the Twenty-fourth Precinct. The cops thought they were cool. They had gone to an emergency room and gotten a tube of surgical gel. While the crew was on a call, they put gel all over the door handles and windshield wipers. They then went upstairs to help, but in reality, it was to give them a legitimate reason for being there when the crew reached for the door handles. Real funny, you might think.

The officers, of course, denied any knowledge of the incident, but their stomach-wrenching laughter betrayed them. The crew took it in stride, accepting it as part of the price they paid working with these cops. Once the patient was delivered safely to the hospital, the crew went into a search and destroy mode.

They found the sector parked on a quiet street several blocks from the Museum of Natural History. The car, its engine running, was parked beside some brownstone buildings. The two officers, male and female, were relaxing. The overhead light in the car silhouetted the two of them.

The driver was reading, as his partner catnapped, thinking of her big date with a male rookie at the station. The EMS crew had been invited earlier to go to a local watering hole to meet the girl and relax with the cops. For this get-together the cop's hair and nails had been done up to perfection. The crew members sought revenge as they inconspicuously rolled up the tree-lined street, pulling abreast of the car.

"Hey guys. What time is the meeting?"

This was just a ploy to have the female cop open her window all the way.

"We get off at one, same as you guys. I guess we should meet at, say, two?" she said, wearily rolling the window down lower.

"Probably a little later," said the tech, not revealing what was about to happen.

"Why? You guys working later?" she asked.

"No, but you will be?" said the tech, smiling.

"Us? No we'll be off."

"No, *you'll* be working."

"What do you mean?" she asked, growing more alert.

"On your hair," said the tech.

She didn't have time to duck as four water-filled gloves were launched inside the car. The first hit her in the head, exploding on her new hairdo. The second ricocheted off her back, knocking the coffee cup and uneaten Chinese food onto her lap. Three and four were the finishing touches. Our fearless crew pulled away to the sound of cursing and the sight of the female officer making unkind gestures ordering them to stop.

The crew members pulled onto Broadway, their dastardly deed done, they smiled. Heading north they sat at a stoplight, the driver glancing in his side view mirror. Suddenly lights appeared behind them. He saw emergency lights from a fast-moving police car darting in and out of traffic. As the emergency lights grew nearer, the siren pierced the night. The crew knew the chase was on!

Up Broadway we, uh I mean, the crew flew in emergency mode, followed closely by the sector from the Twentieth and its soggy, food-covered officers!

Swerving in and out of traffic, the crew headed for the safety of the Twenty-fourth Precinct area, hoping the Twentieth Precinct sector would not follow. But they did. The crew pulled into the Twenty-fourth Precinct and ran inside to the desk sergeant to ask if he had called for a bus.

"I know you too well," said the sergeant. "What are you guys up to?"

"There they are!" screamed the female officer as she and partner stormed through the door. Her hair was in total disarray, adorned with chunks of rice and Chinese vegetables. Coffee and water dripped from her uniform. Her partner didn't fare much better. Everyone got hysterical at the sight.

"We're taking you two out with us!" she screamed.

"Moi? Oh thank you for the offer," said the one tech. "But we really prefer our dates have better personal hygiene."

By now everyone, except the two cops, were howling even a handcuffed perp chuckled. The captain came out to see about the commotion, a dead silence filled the precinct. His eyes shot from the police officers to the EMS crew, and then rested on the police officers.

"I think you should leave now," he bellowed in a no-nonsense voice, freezing everyone in place. "You are out of your sector. You are out of uniform. You are harassing these fine EMS people. And finally, you are dripping . . . what is that . . . on my floor!"

"Yes, sir," the two officers responded.

As they turned, the steam from their anger could have melted an iceberg.

Our heroes turned to the captain.

"Thanks, captain."

"You guys are bad," he said with a broad smile on his face.

"Yes sir. One Four Be Bad Boys, that's us," said the tech as everyone resumed laughing.

The crew did not go to the watering hole that night or respond to jobs in the Twentieth Precinct for a month, always finding a 'flag down' on the street.

**

Vinny and I received a "pediatric cardiac arrest." We pulled up to the building and ran for the elevator. As Vinny pressed the button for the eighteenth floor, a woman got on with two small children. Approaching the floor, I asked the woman to hold the elevator, explaining, "We have a baby in cardiac arrest."

"Shit, I got places to go." she retorted.

"Look, it's a baby."

"Ain't mine!" she yelled, as we got off the elevator running for the apartment. We found the baby in the crib. A neighbor was shouting, "You live in sin. This is your punishment!" Just the type of religious bullshit this devastated mother needed to hear.

I grabbed the kid and ran for the elevator, but it was gone. So we took off, running down eighteen floors. Yes, Vinny kept up, since it was downhill. He carried the equipment while I did mouth-to-mouth and compressions on the kid. As we entered the lobby, Vinny yelled at the cops to grab the mother still upstairs. I jumped into the front seat, as Vinny drove heading to Saint Luke's at One Hundred Fourteenth Street and Amsterdam. All the way, we hoped against hope. All the way, we fought the odds. Vinny called for a standby at the hospital as I continued to do mouth-to-mouth and compressions. The baby didn't make it.

As we stood in the emergency room, an EMS supervisor came in.

"Hurry up. They're holding jobs." Was all he said. Walking outside and before we could even open our sodas

38

we got an "arrest." "No medics were available," so off we went.

The apartment reeked of incense, as two pale, sick-looking police officers dumped coffee grounds on the floor.

"What's up, guys?"

They just pointed.

Viewing the patient, the song "Knock, Knock, Knocking on Heavens Door" came to my mind.

"Okay, it's your turn," I said, turning to Vinny.

"What do you mean?" he asked, confused.

"Hey, I did mouth-to-mouth and compressions on the baby. Now it's your turn."

One of the cops turned colors as we laughed. No need to rush our paperwork now. The patient, she had died in bed several days ago. Meanwhile her playful dog, the one wagging its tail as Vinny petted it, had gotten hungry. Yes, gentle reader, meat is indeed meat.

Three
Justice for Who?

Having never done things in a halfhearted way, I'd reaped both positive and negative results. I'd been fortunate to have a minimal number of negative partners. The following call, and its ensuing disaster, happened with such a partner I hoped to never have again. Here, too, you'll learn of the criminal justice system within EMS that is, itself, criminal.

She was a black paramedic, in more ways than one, senior in patch time, but not street time. The majority of her energy was spent in the "Enchanted Forest," the borough office, rubbing uh... elbows with the chiefs.

Her major problem was twofold in nature. Although highly educated, she could not communicate with people, leading to a history of failed relations. Thus safety and solitude were only found around horses she raised. Standing about five feet eight, she was a strikingly majestic African-American beauty I nicknamed "The African Queen." However, behind fiercely piercing eyes, she had another dark secret. Her skin color was repugnant to her, as confirmed by a black lieutenant I had much respect for T. Hiller on more than one occasion. Working the streets instead of being an awesome role model, she would go out of her way to agitate any Afro-American who called her "sister." The Queen went to great lengths explaining how she was superior to the blacks. Misfortunes stemmed from total insecurity and doubt about who she really was. The Queen, as too many in our world, unfortunately identified herself with skin color, and the insanity was projected to the African-American community, as well as those unfortunate enough to be around her. The "Queen" needed to be "right and white."

One night, we were sitting at Dyckman Street and Broadway. The night had not moved along as rapidly as her mouth. It was her turn to drive and I was a captive audience. Had I been driving, at least I could move the vehicle. But no, instead, I endured the onslaught of her mouth as I prayed for the end of the tour.

Turning my attention to the radio a Harlem BLS (EMS) unit got a job at Post Avenue with a cross of Two Hundred Fourth Street. The job was a 10-90 (unfounded) and the crew returned to Harlem to exchange a portable radio battery on the same radio they were giving the disposition on. I guess someone walked into the dispatch area with food because it flew totally by the dispatcher as to what the crew was pulling.

The dispatcher then called and assigned us an OB (obstetrics) job in the same complex.

We walked into the ground floor apartment to find a young, pregnant female frantically getting her personal items together for her "ride" to the hospital. A young child, grandmother, and brother were present. We asked questions, including if she was high risk or not. She responded no to everything. As the chair was opened, she had a false labor pain, lasting no more than five seconds. I grabbed the drug bag, cardiac monitor, and oxygen bag, as my partner took the patient.

At the bus side door, we had her step up and sit at the end on the bench. It would be easier for her to step off the back of the bus onto a hospital stretcher than be moved stretcher to stretcher. Once vital signs were taken, off we went to the Allen Pavilion, or so I thought.

My partner told the dispatcher she was annoyed at giving the patient a "cab ride" to the hospital. Then she got lost, even though we were two blocks off Broadway. The facility was located at Broadway and Two Hundred Twentieth Street. We had crossed Two Hundred Fourth Street, so the math, as well as the direction to the hospital, was pretty simple. But the mix-up added another five minutes to the ride and five years of stress to my heart. When we finally pulled into the bay, I asked for a stretcher to be brought to the back door of the bus.

Regarding patient care, my philosophy had always been KISS (Keep It Simple Stupid). 'Miss Personality' my partner now walked inside and got into a tiff with both the nursing staff and the doctor. We were quietly waiting in the back of the bus, when the girl started complaining about pain. When I inquired how it felt, she used the key words, "I have to go to the bathroom."

She was moved to the stretcher, stripped, legs were spread to examine her, when I saw a foot. Ah alone with a breach birth, this couldn't get worse could it? You bet your ass it could and did! As I reached with my free hand to open the back door a crack, I inserted my fingers inside the girl's vagina to give the baby a patent airway.

My partner came moseying out, bitching about the staff opening the partially cracked rear door, she froze. For once, something shut this idiot up.

"I need help," was all I said as she turned and walked inside. A few minutes later, a doctor came out and jumped into the back.

"We need help," he bellowed to the nurse behind him.

"I thought you were the cavalry," I said, as we both broke up laughing.

"Keep your fingers in her, while I try to maneuver the kid," he directed.

Shortly the nurse returned with a female pediatrician. "Okay, let's see if we can open her wider. I'll insert my fingers and, Jim, you pull her legs up toward the ceiling."

42

Yeah, seven years in medical school really paid off. Now we had two legs and the butt out. Well at least we knew it was a boy. Being a typical male, this kid did not want to leave the vagina, mother or not.

For the next few minutes I was directed to place this girl in positions one could only find in the Kama Sutra. At least she was flexible.

Meanwhile, my partner was nowhere to be found. "Okay, Jim, I want you to pull as hard as you can, to see if we can get this kid out," the doctor said, as I exchanged positions and body parts with the other doctor.

Continually, through this whole episode I had been talking to the young mother trying to keep her calm. I even had her laughing for a while with my remarks, "Gee, we haven't even had our first kiss yet."

She and the doctors were hysterical. A relaxed body gives. A tense body contracts and tightens. We needed her totally relaxed, to give us all she could, in the way of dilatation. The doctors discussed moving her inside, but they opted to work in the bus. The little lady was starting to tire covered in sweat and becoming scared for her child. She struggled to see how the baby was doing.

The side of the ambulance opened and in stepped my partner, like a prima donna, totally aloof. She took an oxygen mask off the shelf, hooked it into the wall, turned on the oxygen, and waited until the bag was three-quarters full. I glanced over as she placed the mask on the mother's sweat-soaked face. The girl's black hair was a matted, soggy mess. Her brown eyes darted around the ambulance, as she realized her child was in trouble. As she moved her head, the oxygen mask slipped off and hissed as it hit the floor.

My partner, now materializing as 'Miss Compassionate', wiped her hands with alcohol preps, looked at me, and said, "I guess she doesn't want oxygen." Then she exited the vehicle, closing the door behind her!

The male doctor looked at me asking, "What's her problem?"

"It's a long story, starting with her birth."

He chuckled and I thought about the next plan of attack. The infant was out to the shoulders, but we couldn't dislodge the shoulders. I recalled my military training feeling this situation go from SNAFU (Situation Normal All Fucked Up) to FUBAR (Fucked Up Beyond Repair).

We exchanged positions again and I inserted my fingers into her vagina. As the male doctor supported the infant, the female doctor snapped the child's clavicle and I assisted in pulling out the infant. My heart was in my mouth, as we removed the limp infant from the birth canal. The umbilicus was cut, the baby was then whisked into the emergency room, pushing past my useless partner.

She finally meandered over, and we brought the mother in. I checked the infant who was under a lamp, reactive, with good skin color, and breathing on his own.

Between my pass days I had neither seen nor heard anything about my partner or *the call*. Returning to Bellevue, I was told she had been suspended from patient care for the last several days. The other paramedics said she told everyone it was my fault that she was suspended.

"I was only driving. He was in the back," she told anyone within earshot.

So much for this little darling taking responsibility for her overactive mouth and under active assistance on the call. Several days later, I saw her and asked what was up.

"I don't know," she answered nastily.

"Well, would you like me to call and speak on your behalf?"

"Do what you want," she said coldly.

So I called and spoke with doctor, Dr. Macintosh. She pulled the Civilian Complaint Unit letter and read it to me. The doctor who wrote it complained about _my partner's overactive mouth and under active assistance_ and specifically, her attitude. He went on to praise me for my assistance, throwing in numerous accolades. So far so good, right? Wrong. This was NYC EMS.

"Listen, doc, you can't place someone on patient care restriction because of attitude. We would all be out of a job. She has an attitude. But she is a competent medic," I said, really, _really_ reaching.

"Well, the investigation must continue."

After making my phone call in her defense, I read the information faxed to the station. I, too, _now suspended!_ In handling CCUs, EMS policy was to suspend both crew members, no matter what. But I never believe what I see or hear because there is _always_ something deeper behind what appears obvious. Obvious was, the CCU was about my partner. Obvious was, the doctor praised me. Obvious was, mother and child were fine. Obvious to the doctor was the name Schrang. Thus, I was suspended.

We were restricted for the longest time reporting to work in civilian clothes. I cleaned ambulances while she, my darling partner, talked and shuffled papers. If I approached when she was talking to someone, she'd stop, or whisper. Repeatedly, I was told she was blaming me. My response, "It's okay. Time will show her for what she is."

Indeed time does have a way of proving things. Finally, we were ordered to Puzzle Palace, Location One— Headquarters for EMS. We waited in the cafeteria until the CCU investigating officers called us in. I was called in first to meet with two female investigators.

Of all the investigators in the unit, I wound up with former Lieutenant Roberta Post from Bellevue Hospital. She had a less-than-exceptional tour as a paramedic. In one incident she almost got her partner killed. A patient was drowning in the river, her partner dove in. Then she jumped in, unable to swim mind you. He now had two people to save. EMS actually gave this idiot, after she wrote herself up for an award!

So *loved* at Bellevue she had to keep her transfer to CCU under wraps because the crews would have put complaints in against her, thus destroying any chance to get into the unit.

There I sat. "I'm not the primary investigating officer here. I am here to assist this officer," she said. I was grilled by this amateur for quite a while before the "I'm not the primary investigating officer" became the primary investigator.

She asked, "What did you bring with you on the call?"

"Cardiac monitor, drug bag, oxygen, and stair chair."

"Why didn't you bring in the MAST?" (Military Anti-Shock Trousers, used for hypotensive patients, as one example, say, from bleeding.)

"As a paramedic, I can keep her pressure up with fluids (IV large bore). Besides, when was the last time you have ever seen a medic go on an OB call carrying the MAST? To be more specific, when did *you ever* carry them in on a call?"

She didn't like that at all. But she was from my station. Each paramedic makes a name for himself or herself with the EMTs. I had her number, knew her history, and she knew it beyond the 'How stupid can I be in the water' award.

"Explain what happened," she said. I ran through the whole job. Then Lieutenant Post attempted to get cute. In my opinion something she couldn't succeed at on a physical never mind intellectual level.

"So you walked her to the bus."

"No, I told you she was carried out in the chair."

"You said she had oxygen on."

"No, you said that."

"Why no oxygen?"

"Because you were my instructor years ago." Hey, she wants to play games, let the games begin.

"How did she get up into the bus?"

"She stepped up."

"You didn't lift her up?"

"There's nothing in the OPG (Operating Procedure Guide) or better still, medically, why she couldn't step up."

"Where did she sit?"

"On the crew bench."

"Where did you sit?"

"On the stretcher."

"Why?"

"Because it was more comfortable."

"Why are these two blood pressures the same?" She was agitated now.

"Same patient?" I answered with a smile.

"Could you and your partner have lifted the patient out of the ambulance on your stretcher?"

"No, I only had one hand."

Extremely agitated, she asked, "Where was your other hand?"

With this I held up my right hand in front of her face and spread my fingers apart, "In her vagina. Remember, keeping the airway open," I said, wiggling my fingers in front of her.

After regaining her composure, she asked. "Are there any more statements you wish to make? Or questions?"

"Yes."

"Okay. What?"

"I'm an American." Both investigators sat dumbfounded.

"What has that got to do with anything?" Post indignantly asked.

"As an American, I want to know what I am being charged with and by whom."

"I can't tell you that," she said.

"So a criminal will be told these two things, but an EMS paramedic won't?"

"Yes."

The Sixth Amendment of the Constitution of the United States of America states:

"In all criminal prosecutions, the accused shall enjoy the right to a speedy and public trial, by an

impartial jury of the State and district wherein the crime shall have been committed, which district shall have been previously ascertained by law, and to be informed of the nature and cause of the accusation, to be confronted with the witnesses against him, to have compulsory process for obtaining witnesses in his favor, and to have the assistance of counsel for his defense."

So much for that right.

My darling partner was grilled and we returned to the station to continue our exile until ordered to meet Dr. Macintosh who worked for our Medical Director. We finally received orders to report to Puzzle Palace for our audience with the doctor.

Once again, we waited in the cafeteria. This time I did some meditating and actually fell asleep. My partner woke me by shouting my name across the room. We went down a long dreary hallway to a drab room. There was a long table and three chairs with two on one side and one on the other. I couldn't wait for the show to begin.

A male lieutenant from the medical director's office entered first and took a seat.

"These are really serious charges," he said. I guess he was trying to impress himself, because it wasn't working for me. He looked at me and continued, "I hope you realize that after Dr. Macintosh passes judgment, you can be brought up on charges by the chief at your station." I looked at him, then stared, really not giving a damn.

"Schrang, don't you care what's happening here?" he asked.

Before I could answer, my partner started with the tears.

"I care."

I was ready to laugh, but looked at him and said, "Listen. You probably are a nice guy, but three facts remain. First, you're an ass wipe for Macintosh. Secondly, whatever is to be, she has already written in stone. Third, isn't this double jeopardy, allowing us to be brought up on charges administratively after a trial by the Medical Directors Office?"

"No." he said walking out of the room.

So much for the Constitution of the United States, I thought.

Outside, he and Dr. Macintosh had their little talk about the 'unrepentant Schrang'. I would've have loved to have been a fly on the wall.

After the powwow Dr. Macintosh made her grand entrance sporting short hair cut close to the head and dressed in the usual dingy lack-luster gray corduroy pants with plaid shirt, shoulders hunched forward on a six-foot, endomorphic frame. I smiled to myself, thinking she looked like a front-end lineman from the New York Jets.

Without so much as a greeting, she bellowed her first judgment, "I could have sent two MVOs (Motor Vehicle Operators) to do a better job than you two did!"

So much for what the doctor said about my doing a "fantastic job," or for the fact that the CCU *was about my partner*, not me.

So much for being a professional, but my name is Schrang and I had no doubt the 'clique' was targeting me. However, only time would prove this and I was sure I wouldn't be disappointed. This doctor would later have her girlfriend, who was a respected EMS captain, arrested while on duty, in uniform led away in handcuffs for a "lovers' problem." 'Professional? Yeah, my Italian Irish ass!' She unceremoniously plopped down in a chair directly across from us and began a critique of the call and *me*.

"You should have checked for crowning."

I countered that it was inappropriate since the girl did not meet the protocol. NYC EMS Protocol #441 states, **"If mother is in active labor, perform inspection."**

The mother was not in active labor since the contraction lasted less than five seconds. Further it states, **"Contractions must last sixty to ninety seconds in duration and two to three minutes apart."**

Otherwise the patient is having **"false labor pains."** The Brady Book, used by the academy, stated, "If during the physical exam the patient reports the need to push or move bowels, she should be checked for crowning. Examine for crowning only during contraction." Continuing, "Labor consists of uterine contractions that change the dilation of the cervix. Labor is regular and quite painful. False labor is less intense and does not change the cervix."

The meltdown had begun and 'Dr. Bob' did not like the fact that a blind, deaf, or mute person could see this was a hanging and 'Schrang' was not going quietly. I asked her how many babies she had delivered.

"Oh, I saw one delivered in medical school."

My partner chimed in, "I don't deliver people babies. Only horse babies." The idiot makes this statement and the doctor doesn't say a damn thing! See I told you gentle reader I wouldn't be disappointed.

"Well, I stopped counting at just under twenty, with three sets of twins," I continued, "Are you ordering me to spread the legs of every pregnant female?"

"Yes I am," said the doctor.

"Well guess what? I will not," I responded.

It was as if the room suddenly filled with darkening clouds as the egotistical based physician glared. Hunched over the ACR giving a new meaning to 'The Hunchback of Notre Dame' she silently simmered.

With a delivery, one ACR is completed for the mother and one for each of the infants delivered. As a legal document, the ACR must show if any outside assistance was used.

"Your ACRs leave a lot to be desired," she finally snapped.

Before I could say anything the idiot sitting next to me cries out, "Oh, I never saw *his* ACRs."

I looked over at her and said, "Thanks."

My partners, except this idiot and supervisors knew they never had to worry about incomplete or incorrect ACRs with me. I looked at the ACRs. They had the information required, including who was in the back of the bus and the doctor's name. I noted that he was the highest medical authority on the scene. As for the moron sitting next to me....

Finally, the doctor graced us with her decision. We were to report to the Academy for a class and written exam on obstetrics. Also, we were ordered to spend eight hours on an obstetrics ward.

After we returned to Bellevue, Deputy Chief Frederick Villani 'Drop Dead Fred' sent a memo from Luis Matallana, Lieutenant Officer of Medical Affairs, dated 7/11/95. It stated: "The following member(s) of the Service assigned your command have completed the Medical Case Review Process. All patient care issues have been satisfactorily addressed." It listed our titles, names, and shield numbers, and then continued. "All patient care activities have been reinstated. Be advised that no further actions will be conducted through the Office of the Medical Director since our investigation has been concluded. This should in no way negate or influence your individual decision to pursue any independent administrative or disciplinary action. Should you have any questions, please feel free to contact me. Thank you for your anticipated cooperation in this matter."

This was forwarded to: R. McCracken, J. Gombo, P. Carrasquillo, M. Bedell.

The Fifth Amendment to the Constitution of the United States of America: ". . . **Nor shall any person be subject for the same offense to be twice put in jeopardy of life or limb, nor shall be compelled in any criminal case to be a witness against himself . . .**"

How many Constitutional rights had been violated here? Is this a pattern, or is it just me?

We returned to the academy on the specified date. The instructors laughed, as we spent all of twenty minutes with them. Back at Bellevue we were informed the eight hours of overtime on an obstetrics ward had been mysteriously canceled.

But the problems were far from over. Although the CCU was about my partner's mouth and attitude, behind my back, my sweetheart of a partner still told everyone I was to blame for her woes. She talked a lot with 'Drop Dead Fred' who afterwards was of the opinion I had not taken two sets of vital signs on the ACR. Having caught wind of this one day, I approached him as he hibernated in his Bellevue closet, I mean office.

"I understand you don't believe I took a second set of vital signs?"

Confronted in a coffin-sized office, just the two us, with me blocking the only route of escape, he responded as expected.

"Uh, no, I did not state that."

Of course I expected this reaction from him. If he saw something that needed fixing, he found a lieutenant to take action, meaning, "Write that person up." He never had the backbone to take matters into his own hands.

"You had better not, since they were on the ACR," I warned him.

A good example of his failure to have any type of leadership ability or compassion came during a "pediatric cardiac arrest" as was told by Vinny, my friend and now officer. Vinny had a baby in arrest. He sent the EMT outside to retrieve a short board to secure the child. As Vinny worked the baby, he wondered where the EMT was. Finally a fireman brought in the short board, stating the EMT stepped off the curb and had a possible ankle fracture.

Deputy Chief Villani remarked that the EMT's pullover was missing a patch, thus was in violation of the uniform dress code. Next, he went after Vinny and his partner for "being out of service during the re-stock for too long." Vinny re-emphasized that they just had a child in arrest and were taking a few extra minutes to decompress. He told the chief they could either be extended re-stocking for a few more minutes or be put off service by requesting CIS (Crisis Intervention Stress) Team. True to form, the good civilian deputy chief ran off at the mouth. Vinny took it and then told him, "Well, sir, now we are out for the rest of the tour." I taught Vinny well.

The story above gives the picture concerning "Drop Dead Fred." But, where did it all begin? Civilian Deputy Chief Villani and I have a longstanding, warm relationship.

On May 10, 1995, I turned in a "lost and stolen" form after my equipment was destroyed in a car fire. Also, I filed a police report to Lieutenant Espeut, another smooth talking individual with an extremely colorful history that could fill another book. He decides to do a charge package, saying I should have to pay for the equipment. Gee, isn't there something in his background about a large sum of money being stolen, Local 2507, and Mom? What job did she have? Gee, and how was that all resolved? Or perhaps was this payback when one night at the garage Lt. Espeut after a warm and fuzzy discussion outside threatened to shoot me. Yeah, for real I guess I was suppose to show some type of fear because here was a dark skinned man, no cancel that, guy threatening a weapon, but instead told him, "Go for it Eric. Make like a man." He stood there glaring. "Listen," I continued. "I've had real men all over the world try to kill me. Get the fuckin pistol in the car and put it to my head like a man and pull the fuckin trigger." He stood there frozen as his swab debonair façade melted away, turning pasty white. Kind of hard to do when your skin color is of color. When he didn't move, "Oh, that's right, I forgot. Who's going to teach you to take the safety off?" With this he did the smartest thing he ever did around me and walked into the dark night. I always believe if you say something back it up or don't say anything. Thus the charges were forwarded.

Villani wrote, "I concur with Lieutenant Espeut. EMT-P Schrang will reimburse for the replacement of all issued equipment." The document was signed on May 10, 1995.

The next day, I appealed to Civilian Assistant Chief, Manhattan Borough Command, Pedro Carrasquillo. He signed off on it, stating, "Employee to reimburse service for replacement costs." Carrasquillo and Villani snickered when I retorted I would appeal their decisions to Civilian Chief of Field Services Robert McCracken. I was warned, "It won't get overturned in your favor."

On June 26, 1995, I received a letter from Chief McCracken. "Subject: Final Determination—Appeal Approved." When I saw the two civilian gods together they just stared. Assistant Chief Carrasquillo said, "Congratulations, Schrang." Villani chimed in, trying to save face, I'm sure. "Why didn't you tell me you had all this documentation?"

In front of his boss, I said, "Gee, Chief, perhaps you should write yourself up for failure to supervise yourself. You and Espeut had the same material I sent McCracken."

It was a polite way of telling him, in front of his boss, he was both a liar and incompetent. This was the beginning of our warm endearing relationship.

Perhaps years earlier when he was briefly, very briefly on a bus I had met him on the street or on a job and I left a lasting impression. He did not impress me, although he was about to try.

Below is a statement I sent to my attorney as we pieced together the abuse, using documents signed by the parties involved.

On December 16, 1995, my partner Len Swade responded to a call involving a Russian-speaking seventy-two-year-old male. The patient presented with hypertension and chest pain. As we worked on the patient in the back of the bus, another vehicle hit the bus and dragged our vehicle twelve feet. Then the vehicle took off.

There was no major damage; he probably hooked onto our bumper. If there was a scratch, that was a lot. We notified the dispatcher of the situation, including the patient's deteriorating condition. We were told to remain on the scene and await another unit. The nearest unit available was not a paramedic unit and was located at Station Thirteen, East Twenty-sixth Street and First Avenue. We were located at west Sixty-Eighth Street and Amsterdam Avenue; the estimated time of arrival was, minimum, fifteen minutes.

We informed the dispatcher we were going to the nearest hospital because of the patient's condition. We arrived at the hospital and ISU responded along with our patrol boss, Lieutenant Ralph Ortiz. Both agreed we did the right thing in caring for the patient.

In the memo of transmittal, Villani ordered Lieutenant Ortiz to counsel us. Lieutenant Ortiz told him he disagreed with this decision. In Villani's note, he wrote my name first, then my partner's name. On the unit activity log and ACR, Paramedic Swade was listed as driver. Because I was first on his mind, Villani wrote my name first and Chief Pedro Carrasquello signed it, leaving a paper trail.

How refreshing.

The ISU officer, the patrol officer, and the doctors agree we did the correct thing. Villani didn't and ordered the lieutenant to write us up. Whose name is at the top of the hit list, when I wasn't driving? And who backs Villani's decision again? Is it me, or is this a pattern? By the way, does D.C. (Deputy Chief) actually stand for Dumb Choice?

On February 1, 1996, Lieutenant Ortiz issued me a Notice of Counseling. It stated, "You left the scene of a motor vehicle accident involving vehicle 116. You did so without authorization of a supervisor. You are in violation of EMS operating guide procedures," so much for patient care.

Given this historical background, let's get back to the breech birth case. The chief's best shot was yet to come. Charges were filed and on the scheduled day, I reported to the BITS office. My darling partner arrived, bitching and moaning about the lack of parking. Civilian Deputy Chief

Villani entered with his little briefcase in hand. As the door opened, paramedic and friend Tom Reynolds stood beside Don Boyce, one of the legends of One Oh Zebra. He was now a "Judge Woppner" for BITS and would hear my case.

Don looked at Tom, then me, uttering, "What am I going to do with these two?"

Tom and I both smiled sheepishly. There were many very positive things that could be said about Don Boyce. The most important: he was fair and an honest man.

Walking into his office I was ahead of the game realizing he would have to find something to get me on, it's part of the political game. But the punishment would fall far short of what Civilian Deputy Chief EMT Villani wanted—my firing. So I felt pretty good.

Before we started, Don asked if I was willing to accept his judgment as final, or would I go for an appeal. The vice president of Local 2507, Kirk Delnick, objected and told me not to answer. He persisted as I attempted to speak, until I told him to "Shut up". I trusted Mr. Boyce and would accept his decision as final.

As we discussed the case, it was all about me. Don said I should have checked for crowning. I read from the protocol, looking at Villani, and asked, "Are you following this, Fred?" Finally, I stated, "Okay. I accept full responsibility, so let her go."

Of course, the little darling didn't say anything. She sat there, stuck to "Drop Dead Fred."

She and I were asked to wait outside. Suddenly, Villani stormed out of the office, at warp, waddling speed, briefcase in hand. Not even a goodbye! I was truly emotional hurt.

In the end, I lost several vacation days and told of Villani's intent to have me fired, but because of Don Boyce, I was still there. Strike three for "Drop Dead Fred." Oh, concerning my sweet partner, Ester 'C' for '*Can't communicate and Can't take responsibility*' became an EMS Captain and then Deputy Chief from what I was recently told, but if true would you expect less for EMS?

Was this a new experience? Not in the annals of EMS and its tyrannical attempt to rule by fear, intimidation, and violation of Constitutional rights—as the next story shows.

One night, my partner Jack Ng and I responded to backup a crew with a "male shot." The crew that called was a hardworking, competent team, and a pleasure to deal with.

As we approached, the EMT's already had the patient in the back of their unit. My partner walked up to see how things were going, while I got the equipment. Jack asked a housing police officer to step off the bus, while he checked out the patient.

The victim; black male late thirties or early forties. Approaching with the equipment we were informed the shot was to the leg, with an entry, and an exit wound. I got back in our vehicle and waited for the crew to leave as Jack would drop a line (IV) en route to Harlem Hospital, about four blocks away.

We pulled into Harlem and the patient was taken into the trauma room. Once re-stocked and after the crew cleaned up, both units went back into service. This was a typical, uneventful night in Harlem.

Several days later, Jack and I received notification to report to the CCU. No further information was given. Nor did they tell us any other unit was involved.

After wracking our brains, Jack called the Harlem garage and confirmed that the other unit received the same notification. The female EMT informed Jack she urgently needed to talk to us, explaining she had information that couldn't be discussed over the phone. That night we deployed ourselves to the Harlem area to meet with the other unit.

We knew both she and her partner had been in trouble a month prior because they'd called a local TV station about an elderly patient. The crew didn't like the response they'd received after taking the elderly gentleman to the hospital. The social worker had promised to help so long as the crew was there. The following day they were back to pick up the same patient; he'd been released from the hospital without the care the crew sought for the elderly gentleman. The EMS tour commander, a captain, went so far as to threaten charges, telling them, "You're not social workers." A fast phone call from a reporter took care of the matter.

Their 'problem' confirmed what we knew we were working with good people.

The EMT was married to a cop in the Twenty-third Precinct. When she got home the night of the "male shot" incident, her husband said, "Well, do I get my cut?"

"What are you talking about?" she asked.

"You guys ripped off a gunshot victim of several hundred dollars tonight, right?"

"What the hell are you talking about?" she shot back at him.

He laughed, knowing full well she, like 99.9 percent of EMS, was a hardworking Street Saint of Compassion. He filled her in on the rest of the story. Our meeting with this EMT unit was very enlightening.

On the specified day, we reported to Puzzle Palace, Location One, Headquarters at Maspeth, Queens. We waited in the cafeteria on the ground level of Mount Olympus, where the gods resided. Finally, we had an audience with Steve Gilbert, Associate Director, Confidential Complaint Unit, who was the investigator.

Having been asked by popular demand, I took the lead. Walking down the long, depressing hallway, I hung a left, entering a small cluttered office with a smaller room to the side. Inside the small, claustrophobic closet of a room was a bland wooden table and a chair for the investigator. Several feet away, a lone chair with a microphone on an adjustable neck sat. I observed a cheap tape recorder on the table—to be used as a backup, I surmised.

Regrettably, I didn't have my own mini-tape recorder, but the investigation went as follows.

"Your name and shield?" Gilbert stoically commanded.

"Schrang, James M., shield 3257," I answered crisply.

"Do you recognize these ACRs? You are here on a complaint that you or members of the EMS team that worked on Mr. So and So on such and such a date did relieve (rip off) the patient of several hundred dollars. Do you have anything to say?"

"Yes, sir. I do."

"Good, let's hear it." He adjusted the tape to get every word of the kill.

"First, you are the investigator doing this case, correct?"

"Yes, I am."

"Well, I don't know what your credentials are, or even if you have any . . ." Before he could speak, I went on, ". . . but had you done a comprehensive investigation, you would know that this crew is beyond reproach. If you would have done the investigation appropriately, you would know the cop is dirty." He frantically turned off the tape.

"What are you doing?" I asked, raising my voice.

"Uh, that will be all. How did you know?"

"Because I did my investigation. How dare you put us through this crap when you already knew. You owe us an apology."

I was curtly asked to wait outside. Several weeks later we met the crew again. We learned the female EMT got a verbal apology. Needless to say, we didn't and to reiterate this bull shit was nothing new.

After returning from my medical relief missions in Bosnia during the genocide, I was suspended from patient care. To quote Dr. Lorraine Giordano, "I realize you were on vacation, not representing NYC EMS in a foreign land, and people were trying to kill you. But the chief in charge, David Diggs, wants you suspended until you are cleared by the psychiatrists."

I hold the record for the most distant CC (Civilian Complaint) in the history of EMS. An American fireman in

Bosnia, on whom I did a carotid massage with a nine-millimeter in a firefight, wrote a letter of complaint to NYC EMS. Later, I was cleared for EMS patient care. I never received any official apology for being put through hell or regret for character assassination. Nor did I receive an award for my record.

But this begs the question of just how far would Big Brother, in this case now that we were merged with the FD, delve into our private lives?

The First Amendment to the Constitution of the United States of America states:

"Congress shall make no law respecting an establishment of religion, or prohibiting the free exercise thereof, or abridging the freedom of speech, or of the press, or the right of the people peaceably to assemble, and to petition the Government for a redress of grievances."

The Second Amendment:

"The right of the people to be secure in their persons, houses, papers, and effects, against unreasonable searches and seizures, shall not be violated, and no Warrants shall issue, but upon probable cause, supported by Oath or affirmation, and particularly describing the place to be searched, and the persons or things to be searched."

AOL FD style is yet another case of the New York City Fire Department running paranoid. When they learned about www.fdnysucks@aol.com, they wanted to know whose web site it was and who visited the site. Further, they wanted access to the e-mail messages of personnel using AOL claiming they were conducting "an internal investigation of a violation of departmental rules and regulations."

What rules and regulations? I knew plenty of firemen who were anything but team players with the commissioner, yet had their right to free speech been violated by a worthless piece of paper? The Fire Commissioner, Thomas Von Essen, and BITS Assistant Commissioner, Lai Sun Yee, street name

'Dragon Lady,' had enough legal sense to realize no judge would sign their subpoenas.

So being the behemoth of primeval mentality, they decided to use the tactic of intimidation. It worked with AOL, which folded in a New York minute to non-signed subpoenas.

Other more reputable Internet service providers informed Local 2507 they would not honor it. A special thank-you goes to fdnysucks@aol.com for relaying information to me. The results are still pending concerning what the Fire God and Dragon Lady were after, except grief.

We, 'EMS people', don't fold under intimidation.

As an American who was an army paratrooper in Vietnam, I do not appreciate the likes of the Fire God and Dragon Lady who tried to override the Constitutional rights I, and others, have fought for. If the commissioner was investigating criminal activity, why weren't the police notified? Why didn't a judge sign the subpoena?

The civil service weekly newspaper 'Chief' asked the same question. Why were only EMS people targeted and not MetroCare (the mayor's for profit ambulance group) or the voluntary services from the other hospitals or better still firefighters?

To date still no answer, I guess that old saying from Vietnam is true in the case of the Fire God and Dragon Lady. "For those who have fought for it, freedom has a taste the protected shall never know." We, who have served in combat, realize how precious freedom and our Constitution is. Paper- pushing losers, like the Fire God and Dragon Lady, will never understand.

Four
You Want Adult Leadership?
I Think Not!

Giuliani, destruction and paybacks
**We are led by the unknowing, asked to do the impossible,
work with the minimal. And judged by the
unknowing and uncaring.**

The members of the upper crust, the EMS civilian gods, are unique. They range from the extremely talented visionary, ego-hampered 'Big Bird' Chief Paul Maniscalco to the inept and spineless.

However, the ramifications for this festering ineptness by the Rudolph Giuliani administration would affect not only the crews in the streets, but minorities, emergency rooms, clinics, to the most helpless, those in nursing homes. We paramedics and EMT's saw it all as Giuliani micromanaged his surrogates spiraling New York's Health Care System into deeper chaos.

While keeping the spotlight focused on his "war on crime," no one was examining his dismantlement of both Health and Hospitals, the world's largest EMS, and safeguard watch groups. No one cared primarily because it would affect only the minorities.

An aggressive and expensive study by Drs. Jose Sanchez and Jack Kamerman was completed on May 24, 1993, for Health and Hospitals Corporation and Emergency Medical Service. It was undertaken "in response to the deaths of six EMS employees in 1992, three suicidal and three accidental . . . and the role work may have played in their etiology."

Below are three points of interest.

"Paramedics and lieutenants were proportionately more prone to suicidal and par suicidal behavior than other ranks.

"Almost one-fourth of the sample reported feeling burned out. "Given the focus of this research, we sought to understand the relationship between stress on the job and a number of aspects of the work situation. Here again, economic considerations were prominent, as were low levels of support from EMS as an organization and from supervisors, as well as the work itself.

"Among EMTs and paramedics, the focal points of many of their complaints are their immediate supervisors, the lieutenants and captains, under whom they work. The obvious sense of the theme of their criticisms of supervisors, and the vehemence with which those criticisms were always expressed, indicates to us the existence of a real problem that goes beyond the typical carping of subordinates.

One of us witnessed a striking example of supervisory insensitivity. After waiting almost two hours in the emergency room of a hospital for the patient they brought in to be transferred to a hospital stretcher so they could go back into service, a crew member was merely told by the supervisor who had just arrived (presumably to expedite their return to service), 'Why the hell did you bring her to this hospital? No sympathy, no solution, just recriminations.

"EMS supervisors have an 'unwritten' policy of treating people they like one way and people they don't in another . . . [the same] infraction.

They were also accused of expending much of their energy dodging responsibility.

This respondent went on to say that stress results from the CYA (Cover Your Ass) Syndrome so prevalent in EMS. As a result, lieutenants don't take responsibility for even simple decisions. The reality is always there, that in the final analysis the low man will burn."

Below are two of many recommendations of the research.

"Thoroughly review disciplinary procedures. A change that should be considered is that subjects of disciplinary hearings be notified of the charges against them before the hearing. It seems to us that a potential loss of the advantage of surprise is worth the trade-off for the benefits to morale, given the legal guarantees usually taken for granted in a democracy.

"Addressing the critical issues of salaries and benefits would have an impact on a number of stressors in the work lives of EMS employees including: excessive overtime;

"The lack of recognition that EMS workers, by saving lives, do work as valuable as that performed by other uniformed city services; and "The lack of recognition that emergency service work is physically demanding, dangerous, and essential to the public." (Page 101)

It was noted, "Before administering the questionnaire, it was presented to Mr. David Diggs, Director of EMS, and Richard Gutwirth, President of Local 2507—the EMT and paramedic bargaining agent. We secured letters of support from these individuals in order to express to respondents the joint commitment of management and labor to the goal of our study."

Nothing was done with the results of the study. Mr. Diggs was removed after his infamous statement to the New York press concerning:

"Having a plan for a plan in dealing with the snow emergency." This genius became Chief in Charge of Communications, under the fire commissioner. There he was credited with enforcing pressure on dispatchers to turn the mixer off (so units cannot hear each other). The result was civilian deaths in Queens and crews injured by perps with weapons.

Before we were sacrificed to the Fire God, there was a steady trickle of people leaving. In December 2000, there was nothing short of a complete hemorrhage, and nothing was implemented from the study. The chiefs were still the chiefs and the Street Saints of Compassion fought against even greater odds as the Fire God demanded more tours be run with decreasing personnel availability.

As the saying goes, "Shit flows downhill." It flows like one continuous, never-ending, raging river from Puzzle Palace. Let's look at what this rich, shit-filled EMS soil had grown in the way of blooming idiots, I mean leadership.

A story about NYC EMS leadership would never be complete without a few words on such a notable as Lieutenant Paul Giblin, Navy Seal. If you thought Richard Marcinko, who retired _as_ a United States Navy Seal Commander, was a true rogue warrior, you haven't seen anything.

Lieutenant Paul Giblin had a mesomorph frame with some extra fat added on through the years. Yet in build among men, he fit the image of a well-built muscular warrior. I could imagine his large, paw-like hands stealthily paddling himself through the churning South China Sea surf ready to viciously strike. As he deftly left the water his broad shoulders carried those extra pounds of explosives, ammunition for his team, and a wounded swim partner he just saved.

For years he captivated all who would listen with stories of his heroic actions, not only in the jungles and beaches, but also of parachuting into Vietnam. Navy Seals operate in multiple environments.

Paul Giblin, Navy Seal, was attacked by MIG, SAM (Surface to Air Missiles), and antiaircraft flak that filled the skies above Vietnam. Even the Duke, John Wayne, would have been proud to hear of Lieutenant Giblin's combat heroics, like how he broke an ambush by attacking the Viet Cong with his blazing shotgun. I listened in awe to the story of the Navy Seal, who, on one dangerous mission, jumped from a B-52 Stratofortress bomber into Vietnam. Truly, an American hero.

Because of this recognition, he was given the honor of being the patrol boss during Navy Week when his "brothers" conducted airborne and water demonstrations in Manhattan's Hudson River. Many a civilian didn't realize who was in charge of EMS at that event.

Lieutenant Paul Giblin, Navy Seal, matched Hollywood's celluloid expectations of a true warrior. But he lacked two things. Having served as an army paratrooper in Vietnam, I was privy to certain information.

In Jump School at Fort Benning, Georgia, I had my first meeting with the Navy Seals. In any "specialty unit" you learn fast to be the best or be dead. All members of such elite units, no matter what side, are indeed a brotherhood. They have many gifts that drive them to be the very best, but two things are fundamental to all: spine and balls. Lieutenant Paul Giblin, in his everyday actions, demonstrated a complete lack of both.

I never believed he was a Navy Seal. But I also held the conviction that someday it would all come out. Of course, with a little prompting from yours truly, it did. The truth came out one day when real Navy Seals and Army Special Forces rode with us. After talking to one Seal, I introduced him to Lieutenant Paul Giblin, Navy Seal. It took all of thirty seconds for the _real Seal_ to see through Giblin, especially when I reminded him to tell how he jumped out of a B-52 bomber.

The real Seal was sick. He wrote the good lieutenant a note and asked me to deliver it, or he would by pinning it to Giblin's chest, with a knife. I really couldn't afford to stay late on overtime doing the paperwork on how Giblets died so I delivered it before dropping the _real Seal_ at the public library since he refused to ride with the _wannabe Seal._

Later, several Seals wanted to come up and "kick the shit out of some fat lieutenant claiming to be a Seal." Chief Maniscalco (Big Bird) laughingly informed me in Refresher querying, "You didn't by chance have anything to do with this did you?"

On several occasions, Lieutenant Giblin was required to mandate people to fill a vacancy on the tour preceding theirs. If they refused they had to sign a form stating their refusal. This left a paper trail leading to BITS and the Dragon Lady. Our president, Pat Bahnken, wisely put out a directive. We were not to sign anything.

On this particular day there were about four paramedics and an equal number of EMTs in the office with Lieutenant Paul Giblin, Navy Seal. It was a beautiful day and, as such, there were numerous vacancies.

The civilian gods of EMS allowed the Fire God to proclaim proudly to the city council how many tours had been added since the merger. But the numbers did not tell the true story. More tours meant our current workforce of EMTs and paramedics was being run into the ground.

Instead of hiring additional people, they opted to mandate more tours. The gods ordered their henchmen, the lieutenants, to carry out the assignments.

Below is an actual "discussion" by our EMS Navy Seal leader.

"Okay. You people are mandated tonight, since I need the coverage."

"Wait a minute," said Carlos Reyes, "I've already worked a tour this week."

"You have to stay," bellowed the good Seal, getting flustered.

Peter Curry chimed in, "Look, I'm not staying, lieutenant. I've stayed the last three nights."

"I'm leaving," said paramedic Byron Melo, nicknamed the "Colombian Navy Seal."

By God, the crew was abandoning ship! This couldn't happen to Lieutenant Paul Giblin, Navy Seal.

After one outburst, he looked like the wizard from the Wizard of Oz. Remember when Dorothy pulled back the curtain and revealed the real wizard? It was with Lieutenant Paul Giblin, Navy Seal, when the EMTs and paramedics revolted and tore back the curtain revealing the shocked wizard of Battalion Eight.

"You will stay. I'm only following orders," he shouted. "It's not me. I have to follow orders."

Just then the phone rang. It was RCC (Resources Coordination Center, in those days they could).

"Lieutenant Giblin, Battalion Eight."

"Sir, this is EMT so and so. We need a conditions boss (formerly a patrol boss) to run out of Battalion Four."

"I'm not staying," he shrieked into the phone, pulled it to his broad shoulder and looked at us. "You all have to stay." Evidently he heard the voice calling him, so he placed the phone to his ear again.

"Sir, I've been directed by the tour commander to inform you that you are ordered to stay."

"I said I'm not staying. I don't care who says it." He slammed the phone down and looked at us. "What are you laughing at, Schrang?" His face was turning beet red.

"You," Well he did ask right?

"What?" He now jumped up from behind the desk, looking more like a fish out of water than a United States Navy Seal. With flapping arms and jowls in the air, he was in a state of total agitation.

"Paul, watch my lips. You, Y-O-U."

"That's insubordination," he bellowed. The telephone rang again.

"What?" he sounded like a blubbering walrus, not Navy Seal.

I figured it was time to take the lead, since the EMTs were talking among themselves, saying, "Fuck him, I'm not staying."

"I heard that."

"Good night, Paul."

"Where are you going? You can't leave. You didn't sign the paper. I am only following orders."

Being a military man, he seems to have forgotten another group of clowns who said the same thing in Germany.

"Paul, listen closely. I'm not signing anything. Nothing, zip." The lower and more calmly I spoke, the more he went into a state of panic.

Storming from behind the desk he moved to the cabinet. My partner cranked him even more.

"The captain told me to get a second job, so that's what I did. I'm not staying. I don't want to be late for it."

The phone rang again.

"Don't answer that!" he shrieked.

Upon opening the cabinet, he found only one form for the eight of us.

"Good night, Paul," I said heading for the door, knowing others would follow.

"Wait, Schrang! You have to sign. I'll make copies."

"Paul?"

"Yes?" he probably figured the threat worked.

"Paul. If I wait for you to make copies of the form, I'll refuse to sign. But you'll have to sign."

"Me?"

"Yes, Paul, you. You will have to sign my overtime sheet for the time I stayed here waiting for you to make copies of a form I'm not signing.

I don't think the captain will like that. Good night."

There was a mass exodus out of the office, while he made copies that no one would have signed. No one stayed. Talk about leadership by example.

As we filed out of the door, Lieutenant T. Hiller smirked and shook his head. He was a black officer and gentleman, who always led by example and was approachable. He actively sought solutions with the people under his command. This was in contrast to the majority who sought no solution. They only inflamed the problems.

A fire was raging in a tenement apartment. The workers had been stripping the floors with a highly combustible solvent when one of them lit a cigarette, proving once again, smoking can be hazardous to your health.

We pulled in behind, keeping our distance from the EMS command vehicle. Lieutenant Paul Giblin, Navy Seal, and Mike Phillips were riding together. Lieutenant Giblin, being the senior officer, wanted to show the new lieutenant how operations in the field were supposed to be conducted.

"Paul, you can't park here," Lieutenant Phillips said to Lieutenant Giblin, who was driving.

"I'm here. The fire is there. Why not?"

"Because that is the fire, those are the fire trucks, and you are parked in front of the fire hydrant. That's why!" With this, a mentally weary Lieutenant Philips exited the vehicle.

The EMTs pulled up behind us as the smoke billowed out of the second-floor apartment, firemen ran in their hoses in hand. The sidewalks were crowded with people watching the operation. Lt. Phillips had us hysterical telling us about riding with 'The Navy Seal'. Suddenly our laughter turned to panic as the emotionally frustrated 'Seal' floored the accelerator. The command vehicle lurched onto the street and into the path of a fast-moving fire engine and crew. With siren blaring, the engine chauffeur frantically locked up the brakes, shrouding us in smoke as the engine swerved out of control in our direction. The chauffeur's eyes filled with terror as firemen in the cab screamed. We dove for cover behind our vehicles as civilians ran screaming in all directions. After the brake smoke cleared, we peered over the hoods of our vehicles in total awe. The engine had missed our unit by a foot ending its uncontrolled death slide about ten feet from a ladder truck. We looked over to see the oblivious Lieutenant Paul Giblin, Navy Seal, parking his vehicle across the street, blocking yet *another fire hydrant*.

We went to work as a burn patient was brought to us while Lieutenant Phillips went over to yell at Lieutenant Giblin, Navy Seal, the senior officer in charge.

According to the operating guide, a patrol supervisor is on the scene to ensure things run smoothly and to be an administrative asset to the crew. If we had multiple trauma patients, the patrol boss alerted us as to the available trauma and the number of burn beds available. However, the final word on definitive care still rests with the paramedic. In this situation we just wanted to clear the scene fast! Thus the EMTs begged us to place the patient in their bus and we, the paramedics by working in their bus, would insure both units could leave...fast.

A less dramatic case took place with my buddy, Lieutenant Paul Giblin. We had just finished a "cardiac arrest" and returned to Battalion Eight to re-stock and clean up. Tom Reynolds had gone to the sink to rinse out the suction unit, only to find the drain clogged. He went to use the sink in the bathroom.

Lieutenant Giblin was on patrol, seeing Tommy, yelled not to clean the suction unit in the sink.

We had an EMT I'll call "Useless," since his job was to have clean suction units as well as other equipment ready for the crews. Needless to say, this didn't happen. Thus, we had a problem. We couldn't go out without portable suction. Tom and I walked into the office. A lieutenant and several EMTs were there.

"Excuse me, Lieutenant Giblin," I said.

"What?" he bellowed.

"First, what are we to do about this suction unit? Secondly, you should watch how you speak to people."

"I don't care what you do with it. But you will not wash it in that bathroom," he said, getting flustered.

"Listen. We are seeking a solution from you, a supervisor. We do not want nor expect you to add to the problem. Now I'll ask again. What can we do about this dirty suction unit?"

He hollered and everyone in the room started smiling, "Schrang, get out of here!"

"Not a very friendly approach, Paul. Remember what I said about watching the way you talk to people?" Now he was really cranked.

"I'm giving you a direct order. Get out!" That did it.

"Direct Order like, Navy Seal, right? Paul, you and I both know you were never a Navy Seal. You *were* a radio repairman and you *sucked at that too*...right?"

Now he ran around the office as everyone laughed at him. Sitting down, he bellowed, "This is insubordination. I'll tell the captain. Get out." Now that was a real mature way of handling it.

"Paul? Paul?" Everyone became quiet as Tom stood there, with the suction unit dripping vomit on the floor. "Paul?" He looked at me, as he grabbed his chest. "Is the pain bad yet? Is it radiating to your arm?"

"Get out! I said get out!"

"Paul, you're turning red. I'm asking because I care and I'm waiting for you to go into arrest."

"Get out, Schrang." Everyone in the office was rolling.

"Paul? When you do go into arrest, no one, but no one, except for me, will work on you."

"Schrang! Everyone get out. I don't want you working on me."

Of course, no one left. More crews walked in to see about the commotion.

"But Paul, I care. Plus, I want you to wake up intubated." He looked at me.

"Yeah?" he said for the first time without bellowing.

"Yes, I do. That's so I can do to you, what I would do for my three favorite people."

"What?" he asked.

"I want you to open your eyes while intubated, just like in my dreams of Mayor Koch and Jane Fonda. Yeah, and when you open your eyes I want you, and them, to see me piss down the tube."

He lunged from the table, shrieking my name.

Everyone was hysterical. Tom and I left never receiving help for our problem we finished washing the suction unit in the "Paul Giblin, Navy Seal, Memorial Shitter." Later he waddled from the office heading to the lieutenant's office to write me up on charges. I stood there whistling "Anchors Aweigh," the U.S. Navy anthem.

Paul Giblin was basically harmless, and did not have a mean or vindictive streak in him, much like Sgt. Schultz on

Hogan's Heroes. That could not be said for others who relished making others a personification of the living hell their own personality of self reflected, and in one case ending it.

I met one EMT who attempted to hang himself at Battalion Twenty-six, because of a lieutenant. The only reason the man is alive is because the rope broke.

According to the people I interviewed, the lieutenant had unmercifully harassed the EMT. The lieutenant didn't have any particular reason while the EMT sought understanding and sympathy from others at the station.

Wasn't it strange that the one being harassed was seeking to understand?

Yet the lieutenant, the boss, the instigator, did not. Instead he chose to inflame the problem, not be the source of a solution.

Another case concerned an EMT from another Bronx battalion who sought help when he needed time off because of marital problems. He was told by the supervisor, "If I was married to you, I'd divorce you also."

The EMT went home and shot to death his wife, then himself, reportedly in front of their young children.

But this uncaring ineptness was not only endemic to supervisors directly above the EMTs and paramedics. It was rampant up the chain of command.

On September 19, 2000, I had a problem, once again, with my partner Guy Grillo as had our partner paramedic Arty Gonzales. Grillo had a pattern of having problems. He was an angry young man who lacked the ability to deal with his frustrations on the job. As noted by several people through the years, his anger had grown, as had the frequency of his confrontations with partners. Captain Mark Stone, then Battalion 8's CO, urged me to write him up. Grillo had the problem first with Arty and he, Grillo was detailed to the Bronx, Arty remained at the station. When Grillo had the problem with me, I followed Captains Stone's orders, wrote him up and we were _both_ promptly transferred to the Bronx. DAH, did I miss something here?

One of the things I'd learned was to accept. It didn't mean I let people walk all over me. Rather, I picked the time and place to voice my opinion.

Chief Frances Pascale 'Ole Kneepads'(Bronx Command) graciously did her best to keep me on a morning-to-afternoon shift of tour two. For this, I was grateful.

On September 27, 2000, after being jerked around by Captain Stone, I talked with Lieutenants Ricardo Mercado and Giuseppe Lavore and put in for a transfer to remain on Two-six Willie with Angelo Morales. All showed concern and helped me make the decision. To all, I am grateful.

The reaction was utter disbelief. One EMT told me the captain was furious saying "How can he transfer when he was sent there as a punishment and on top of that he likes the South Bronx better than Manhattan!" Gee I was happy to make his day.

During the course of the day, I had the pleasure of taking care of Captain Medinas's mother. His parting words to me were, "I hope they don't screw you now that you want to stay." He was one of the best.

I arrived home to find a certified receipt from the post office from the fire department. Needless to say, I wouldn't sign for it. They know where I work.

Several days later I called Captain Stone to ask what was happening with my transfer.

"I don't know, since I'm out of the loop on this. I haven't spoken to the chief, so I don't know."

"No, you are not out of the loop, because I did as you said and was detailed."

Silence, sad but true. Captain Mark Stone had much ability. Unlike Chief Maniscalco, it wasn't an ego problem, it involved the spine.

"I will not go out on a limb for anyone at this station if it will endanger my chances of becoming chief." Stone told me once and in this case he kept his word.

To add a final note and show you how much the captain lived by this motto, EMT Gus Blanco, known as "Switch Blade," returned to Battalion Eight one day after leaving BHS prior to my being 'detailed'. Gus Blanco was a burly five-foot-eight-inch-tall Hispanic. Gray hair and mustache were accented by glasses that sat on the top of a well defined pug nose, cigarette from his mouth. His potbelly girth was more representative of an oversized Puerto Rican leprechaun, than the "strike macho woman's man" he loved to be thought of as.

Gus had been short of breath and he visited the FD doctors at BHS, who told him, "Here's your EKG, go see your own doctor." The doctor coolly responded, wanting him to leave the grounds immediately.

"By the way, you are suspended patient care. One more thing," he continued, not looking up from his computerized list, "Oh, you're EMS, not a firefighter; if you have no sick time or annual leave, no paycheck."

EMTs and paramedics have a physically taxing job, but no heart bill. Gus looked concerned and confused as he entered Captain Stone's office.

Shortly, Captain Stone stormed out, extremely upset, leaving Switch Blade inside. Gus called me to take a look at his EKG. As we stood in the captain's office I explained the EKG. The signature easy Hispanic smile was gone, replaced by the face of a man having heard his death sentence. With no coverage, no paycheck meant no support for his family.

Captain Stone came in, yelling at both of us, "Get out of my office!"

"Did you see this EKG?" I asked.

"Yes, I did," replied the captain who is a "book only" paramedic. He was one of the few who took the medic program when the fire gods decided only paramedics could be officers, but even Howard Sickles didn't complete the actual hours needed for the patch. But that's another little dirty secret. Captain Sickles would try to fly with "Well I'm a paramedic with Hatzoloh" but would become infuriated when paramedics who knew the deal asked him "So how long are you going to remain a junior (new) medic?"

But let us get back to Gus. "It's not my responsibility," captain Stone barked, looking at the EKG.

"Well, as a medic, I would not be allowed to leave a patient like this," I replied.

"You are not a doctor. Now leave."

We went into the lounge and I explained the strip to Gus.

"Hey, why don't we get you in down the hall, here at Bellevue?" I asked.

He wasn't too keen on the idea, but was still open to suggestions.

"Okay, how about if I get a medic unit back, or pull my stuff out of the storage locker?" He was still open.

I walked into the main office and said to Captain Stone, "Sir, how about you talk to him about getting checked in the ER?"

"He is not my responsibility!"

"Okay, how about I work him?"

"You are an EMT." (I was working with an EMT that day. I was not allowed to do Advanced Life Support, since there must be two medics.)

"How about I call a medic unit back then?"

He looked at me his eyes flashing, "No! He is not my responsibility and I want him off the grounds."

I walked inside, really pissed, and told Gus. He took it in stride and said the captain flipped out when he realized he would be short by an MERV operator and had to place someone on overtime. It messed up his statistics for the chief.

A leader must take responsibility for his people. The Caregivers take care of everyone, every time, no questions asked. Yet when we needed to take care, we got "Not my responsibility" from the supervision, especially a captain.

Gus had a touchy bypass surgery and returned to work, no thanks to EMS supervision, a gutless captain who would go on to become an EMS Chief, Is it me or are we seeing a pattern here?

One final note concerning caring leaders to provide balance demonstrating not all supervisors or doctors were like Mark Stone and the FDNY doctors. Dr. William Motley was the medical director in 1992. He was a true paramedic's doctor.

More than once, he showed up on the scene, instilling confidence in the paramedics. He was sincere and caring. If we were hurt, he would be there, checking on us 24-7. He didn't fit the mold, so he was ushered out the door and no medical director since has held a candle to him.

Two other notables in the ranks were Captain Ellen Shibelli and Lieutenant Roy David. On two separate occasions each sent a sick member home with no questions asked. Lieutenant David embarrassed our Navy Seal to call RCC, so the member could be driven home, instead of taking public transportation. These were the bosses I would go the extra mile for any day. Unfortunately, these days of FD micromanagement, one would need to travel more than a mile to find such leaders.

There was an extremely young morbidly obese lieutenant at an EMS station who relished his manipulation of people, as much as he relished his cigars. I won't use his name to protect the lieutenant you'll read about that we all admired. While awaiting his captain's bars, this was the way he got his jollies, second only after manipulating his favorite female lieutenant.

This lad was recently married to a doctor, but had perverted urges. He stole away with said female lieutenant in the captain's office hour after hour. This created major problems. The female lieutenant was married and greatly respected.

Often the two lieutenants were in the captain's office "talking" and no one was allowed in. Crews sat and waited while the two finished their "talk."

When the lieutenant left for the day, he'd call the garage to continue the talk. This loser even bragged about the expensive jewelry he bought her in New Jersey, showing it to a certain paramedic. She on the other hand was warned by concerned crews that the situation didn't look right and would end in a homicide if her husband found out.

One day there was a buzz at the station after a number of people saw her interviewed at a New Jersey mall. Jewelry from Jersey, he lived in Jersey, she didn't, and now in an interview from a New Jersey mall.

Finally, she wisely transferred out.

This same male, the executive officer of Battalion 8, under Captain Mark Stone's Command, had an even darker demonic side. Because of his weight he probably had poor self-esteem, which translated into receiving sordid pleasure out of other people's grief.

At the station, he had a little clique of EMT's. One of the games they played was to have a new EMT strapped to the long board and hosed down. One day, while he was behind the desk, he watched, chomping on a cigar, as his raiders went after a tall, thin EMT. The crew stripped the EMT naked, secured him to the board, and then measured his penis. They all, including this officer, had a good laugh. The kid went home crying.

Do you think the captain of the station upon learning about what happened and did anything? Yeah, if you believe that then you'll believe President Clinton didn't have sex and George W. can complete two sentences without embarrassing the nation. The EMT became a paramedic and changed boroughs. This dysfunctional lecher was promoted to captain, who loves computers and cigars;then Deputy Chief…would you expect less? Please note the only reason I didn't give his name was to protect both the female officer's marital status and the EMT.

NYC EMS under FDNY tyrannical micro-management had turned into a deadly toxic environment, a true cesspool of despair for the human mind. EMS leadership was always reactionary, never visionary. They waited for something to happen before they reacted. Now that they were forced to run more tours with fewer resources to satisfy the phony statistics lauded by their FD masters of the Giuliani administration, the stress increased.

Thus, the EMS system, which had the most calls in the world, for so long led by ineptness that bordered on stupidity, started to buckle.

The following story shows how they ruled by fear and fostered pain— their own, yet managed never to learn anything.

He had worked for NYC EMS in an "upper" supervisory "suit" position and left to run a mid-sized town's EMS. The year had been very productive and he relished his success. He decided to have a pool party at his home and invite the crews as well as others.

The party was going very well. It appeared everyone was having a great time. The pool was adorned with bikini-clad EMTs and paramedics who worked for his startup ambulance service. Life was good, he thought, looking out over his little kingdom.

The aroma of the grilled hamburgers and hot dogs filled the air, accompanied by the sound of beer cans being popped open. The white foam exploded skyward and onto some swim suited guest. Everyone had a good time as the music blared on this hot August day.

He decided to have a contest. The winner would receive twenty-five dollars. The three most beautiful workers were picked. The contest began.

"If you take off the top of your bikini, you will win twenty-five dollars."

Everyone cheered as the three girls laughed and giggled.

"Come on. Who is going to be the winner?" he asked, holding up his beer as the cheers grew louder.

The girls looked at one another, each coaxing the other on. Finally, one girl reached behind her back and took off her top. Holding it in one hand she lowered it to her side. There she stood, a true goddess, the winner.

The crowd roared. She stood there with succulent breasts exposed for all to enjoy. He walked up to the winner, gave her the twenty-five dollars, and got a kiss, a kiss of death.

The rest of the night continued uneventfully. Well after dark, everyone drifted home. A fantastic time was had by all at the boss's house.

As he sat on the porch under the star-filled sky he smiled, feeling content with himself. It had been the best Saturday of his life.

Monday morning at his office he was served. In a lawsuit that followed, the girl who removed her top said she felt "pressured" to remove her clothing, since he was the boss. He lost the business and his were dreams crushed, as she was rewarded much more than twenty-five dollars.

Now, having heard such a story, you'd think FDNY EMS supervisors would take the hint. In the above story, the other two girls had the same boss and decided not to remove their tops. The majority of his workforce liked him, and he had felt comfortable enough to invite them to his home.

This was not the case in FDNY EMS, where chiefs wouldn't even bring their personal cars near where they worked. Here the majority of the workforce despised the supervisors. One would also think that the episode of Pizza Man and the EMT would have caught their attention to the problems of sex in the work place. One female paramedic won over a million dollars after she was wired by NYPD after numerous sexual assaults. So you'd think these people would have learned. Wrong.

EMS Station Eleven was the Borough Command (The Enchanted Forest) in lower Manhattan. A supervisor was leaving EMS so the commanding officer and other officers were present when the "going away gift" arrived—a stripper. But not just any stripper, a male stripper, for the male lieutenant. Everybody had fun as the "gift" unwrapped. However, there was a problem.

The supervisors went out of their way to make life difficult for the crews. In one incident they got up on the wrong side of the bed, thus changed the schedule, resulting in destroying the crews' home lives. The harassment was hot and heavy. The supervisors followed the policy of rule by fear. If there was a way to help a member and make things easy, they did the opposite.

The payback came when a male EMT put in a sexual EEO complaint *with video*. BITS was called in, the officers in question were untouched retained there jobs and fined. As for the video...I have often stated time and again that what one projects will come back to oneself multiplied. Here once again my brothers and sisters proved me correct in their response to an ego-ridden; intellectually challenged group of dysfunctional bosses.

Unlike Battalion Eight in midtown Manhattan, Battalion Twenty-six was deep in the South Bronx, where things were different. The borough had the worst hospitals in the city. Jacobi Hospital had been heralded as the Mecca of knowledge. In my humble opinion, Jacobi and its nursing staff couldn't hold a candle to King's County Hospital on a bad day or to Bellevue Hospital on its best day.

Saint Barnabas Hospital was another example of how Mayor Giuliani had hurt the minorities of this city with his payoff to MetroCare Ambulance.

It was the for-profit ambulance service given the green light by the Giuliani *after* the corporation contributed to his election campaign.

Where was the city council speaker, Vallone, or Bronx borough president, Ferrer, when others asked about MetroCare's reported $400,000 payment in penalties to U.S. Health Care Financing Administration for improper billing, overbilling, and unnecessary ambulance rides? It was reported that MetroCare overbilled Medicare to the tune of $4.8 million. Where was everyone?

MetroCare operated out of Saint Barnabas and was a disgrace. I witnessed a young Cambodian child brought in with positive loss of consciousness and nausea from a fall.

The child, without even the correct neck collar on or secured to the long board appropriately, should have been taken to a Trauma Center but instead was brought to Saint Barnabas.

This was not good patient care, but rather, steering, which is when you disregard the patient's needs and bringing the patient to your hospital, regardless of his/her condition—which boiled down to making money, not patient care. I looked at the MetroCare crew and realized that the potential was great if I ever left FDEMS to work there to teach what I had learned, if their management was interested.

Saint Barnabas itself could do no wrong. EMS chiefs stood silently by as FDNY had one FDNY paramedic fired and another brought up on charges for taking a non-critical asthma patient to Jacobi instead of Saint Barnabas. The patient had a Jacobi card and had been treated at *both* hospitals. When she later returned to Barnabas, she informed the staff she had been taken to Jacobi by FDNY. The Fire God had the paramedic fired. The man found out he had been fired while at home with his wife, watching TV.

Then the Gestapo, BITS, launched their henchmen into every emergency room in the city. They'd ask the patient if this was really the hospital he wanted to go to. Once again EMS civilian chiefs did not give a shit about the fact that the crews did the right thing. They wanted to undermine the public trust of the crews and appease the micromanaging, egotistical Giuliani administration.

The crew in question did nothing wrong. Yet, it cost one man his job, because a hospital administrator complained. Once again the chiefs acted true to form. Later, much later he would be hired back but only *after signing a waiver so he wouldn't sue FDNY!* If, FDNY had nothing to hide, why the waiver?

At the same hospital, there was a twenty-two-year-old Ecuadorian female who walked into the mirror of a truck as it started turning from a dead stop. The mirror was intact and there was no trauma to the patient, other than her left facial cheek hurt. The BLS (EMTs) brought her to Saint Barnabas Hospital. The nurse shouted, "trauma notification!"

The crew was in shock. The doctors came running. As the staff forcibly stripped the protesting girl, the female crew member yelled,

"What the hell are you doing? It's not a trauma notification!"

The girl did not meet trauma criteria. But because Saint Barnabas wanted to be a level one Trauma Center, they mistreated the girl, to increase their statistics for the state evaluator. Hey Trauma Center equals more status, more money. The girl was stripped naked and had a finger put up her ass, checking for occult bleeding. This was nothing less than legalized abuse of a patient to build up statistics, a violation of a minority girl who trusted the medical staff. But there was someone in the wings that could and would make a difference.

Another hellhole was Bronx Lebanon Hospital. It had two divisions. In the Fulton Division I was educated only to bring EDPs (Extremely Disturbed People) and drunks. There are no words to describe this place.

At one point it was closed to 911 units because the "doctors" could not even intubate patients! Bringing in a drunk, you would have to navigate, then, compete for the nurses' attention while a fistfight broke out in the waiting room. The Concourse Branch was even deadlier.

A forty-year-old Jamaican Rastafarian gentleman lost his leg up to the hip. Why? He had a clot in his lower leg. Somehow the incision didn't heal. It wasn't dealt with in a timely manner and an infection spread until his entire leg had to be removed. I had no knowledge of his medical records, but after listening to him and his wife, I would just about guarantee this would have never happened at Bellevue.

One night, we brought in an APE who was dying. We had called ahead with a notification. Yet when we arrived, no stretcher, no respirator, and the medical team stood around with their fingers up their asses. Instead of saving this woman, we contributed to her death by bringing her to this inept staff.

Although the staff, in particular certain nurses at Bellevue, bitched up a storm when Dr. Goldfrank was in the emergency room, we got results. After witnessing what happens inside these South Bronx emergency rooms, I appreciated Dr. Goldfrank more than ever. Bellevue Hospital was, without a shadow of a doubt, the premiere emergency room others could only hope to emulate.

Dr. Goldfrank was an exacting taskmaster and not one of my three favorite doctors, but he demanded excellence, and the results spoke for themselves. Years ago, this statement was attributed to him: "You could train a monkey to do what paramedics do."

When we heard this, it pissed us off. As for me I set out to show him and, through the years, worked hard to be as good a paramedic as possible. I had an obligation to paramedics like William Simon, Jack Ng, and Lori Santo who believed in me.

Evidently, I was not alone. During an interview years later, Dr. Goldfrank told a reporter, "Years ago, people would ask, 'Is there a doctor in the house?' Today you had better ask, 'Is there a paramedic in the house?'"

This sentiment of professional recognition would be echoed within the Bosnian Mission of the United Nations where I went years later to assist their civilians during the genocide.

The interview bolted like lightning through the Bellevue EMS garage. There were a lot of smiles that day, realizing we had shown this renowned doctor something. But in my heart, I believe he was asking us to come up to his standards. In the end, we all were winners: the paramedics, Bellevue Hospital, but most of all, the patients. In this regard, the hospitals in the Bronx were not even in the same universe.

There are *several disadvantages* I found endemic to the Bronx, in particular, the South Bronx. *First*, the majority of people come from third world countries where a doctor is not questioned. Thus, on more than one occasion, I would ask a patient what he or she was allergic to and be told, say, aspirin as an example. Holding up the bottle containing the medication, I'd ask, "Well, if you are allergic, why are you taking it?" The response,

"My doctor said take it."

Second, most doctors I met in the South Bronx were practitioners, not healers, and were only concerned with the Medicaid, Medicare card for payment and their over inflated egos. On too numerous occasions we responded to "asthma" calls where the child had not been treated at all but the nurse informed us the doctor was demanding the patient be sent to his hospital! Talk about steering and manipulation of funds.

My partner and friend paramedic Angelo Morales was sitting at a fire scene on the corner of Southern Boulevard and Westchester Avenue when a woman came hopping over to us. "Did this happen during the fire?" we asked examining her ankle.

"Oh no," she answered, grimacing in pain. "The doctor in the San Juan Clinic (directly across the street) saw you guys and said for me to get to the ambulance before you left."

Extremely pissed, I asked, "Did he take your Medicaid information?"

"Yes," she replied innocently, suddenly realizing the point we were making.

So how was it that these charlatans calling themselves doctors were allowed to prey on these people? This was the ***third*** problem.

These "professionals" benefited from the decision in 1999 by our "great Law and Order Mayor" to abolish the 911 Committee, which served as a watchdog for just such problems. The Committee bought together representatives from emergency rooms in the city as well as EMS and could force emergency rooms to upgrade to the committee's standards.

According to New York City Comptroller Alan G. Hevesi, "The professionals on the 911 Committee brought about a quiet revolution in emergency room care in the '80s and early '90s, turning emergency rooms from dumping grounds for incompetent physicians and moonlighting interns into professional operations."

Thus without this watchdog group, the weakest population, the minorities of the South Bronx, would be abused even more.

The *fourth* was that of discrimination politically, even by *their* elected officials. Several years ago, some firemen got into a fight in a bar. They did some damage and were arrested. The Fire God said, "It's under investigation."

Several weeks later, a young female, nine months pregnant, had an asthma attack in the South Bronx. She went into cardiac arrest. An EMS paramedic unit was sent from Harlem. Several times, they asked for backup, as well as directions, since the street location was not on their maps. The woman and her baby died.

I lost all respect for the Bronx borough president when the headlines from the Fire God read, "EMS Messed Up." Mr. Ferrerr should have been screaming for the answer to the question: Why wasn't a fire department truck dispatched immediately?

I'll tell you why. It was the South Bronx, not Midtown Manhattan. It would have never happened in Manhattan. There would be too many whites, too many lawyers, too many cameras, and we all know how the fire department loves cameras.

Thus during this period of time our local (2507) cried out and squandered resources on losing litigation against MetroCare. It is one thing if you win, but this was not happening. It is my humble opinion that all of us and the public we serve would have fared better if the union officials worked *with* the MetroCare personnel via training courses, and dramatized the loss of this mother and child showing the correlation with the Mayor's destruction of the 911 Committee through educational town meetings, press releases, etc.

Instead the union got everyone up in arms about the *for profit* company yet failing to mention that the only reason EMS was given to FDNY was because as a political payoff it was a cash cow. To reiterate, when a fire engine responds to a house fire *you don't get billed*. When the police respond you *don't get billed*. But when EMS responds, well **it's all about the money.**

Another place the crews loved was the Daughters of Jacob Nursing Home. But exactly what is a Nursing Home according to the Public Health Law in New York? According to this law, "Public Health Law classifies nursing homes as hospitals." EMTs and paramedics hated nursing homes. I have yet to see one I want to die in. Yet this was where many families dump their parents to die. It was a cold, but true, statement of the "Me" generation. What we experienced were out of sight, out of mind hell holes.

This home — pardon me, hospital — typified too many and was known by the crews as "Daughters of Death." We had one job where the doctor wanted the patient taken to the hospital because her "breath sounds were shallow." The patient was on a respirator! It, not the patient, was breathing. As the doctor listened, one of the crew members reached over and turned the respirator knob controlling the volume. The doctor looked up.

"Gee, doc, how are her lung sounds now?" the medic asked.

"Oh much better, but I want her out of here, so the emergency room staff can figure this out."

"Good idea, doctor," the medic's partner said with a smile, at the incompetent physician.

The EMTs rolled their eyes. But trust me the Daughters of Jacob were not the only ones who deserved such recognition as you'll read below but first let's revisit Daughters of Death.

On another trip to *Daughters of Death*, my partner and friend, paramedic Brian Sparbar, and I responded to a "cardiac." We found the patient sitting in a wheelchair in an office. Two people were sitting with him; neither was a nurse or doctor.

Approaching the patient, he informed me he had been having chest pains for the last hour and his arm was going numb. During this period of time, neither person so much as moved to call for a doctor.

I attempted to check the man's pulse, only to find he did not have one. I rapidly checked the other wrist and he had one. I attempted a blood pressure reading in both arms. There was none I could detect while asking Brian to confirm my find, which he did. As far as we were concerned, everything else could be done en route.

We started the workup after the patient was loaded into the back of the bus, calling for a notification with surgical consult at Lincoln Hospital.

Once there the gentleman thanked us as he was rushed upstairs to have a surgical procedure to save his arm and life. Lincoln had come through. The same could not be said concerning the two losers we met.

About a month after receiving the thanks of the doctors and the patient, we were called into our captain's office. Captain Andy Werner had received a CC from one of the parties. It seemed the EMS gods wanted answers, fast.

I learned that the complaint was from a social worker who was upset on three counts. *First*, no one had spoken to her. *Next*, the crew did not take the wheelchair with them. How was the patient to come home? *Finally*, no one asked her anything.

From my point of view, the patient was talking and critical. He was in a medical facility, using this term loosely. The social worker did not call for "medical professionals", then complained we did not talk to her. This idiot did not even have the common sense to have a copy of the patient's chart waiting for us. I had to find that information in route…from the patient!

I submitted my first statement to the captain. We had been blessed to receive Andy Werner as our captain, and Carl Tramontana as our deputy chief. In this case, DC did not stand for dumb choice.

The next day, Brian and I were called in to "rewrite" our statements. We rewrote our statements to be more politically correct, to save the new captain's ass. The chief got hysterical when he read the originals, as the captain shredded them in front of us, his chest pain decreased with each shredding. Another lesson in the lack of leadership, not these two, but the losers in EMS Bronx Command who kissed the asses of people like our little social worker.

An article in the Daily News dated January 15, 2001, reported that of seven people who died in the Meadow Park Nursing Home, not one had been given CPR. By definition, CPR is a means of sustaining life when the heart and breathing stop.

The state investigator asked the nurses about CPR and made an interesting observation. He asked one nurse when CPR should be given. She answered it should be done when residents are choking. Another said it should be started when the resident has labored breathing and a rapid pulse. Both answers were incorrect. The report stated that "significant corrections" were warranted at Meadow Park and Bezalel Nursing Home in Far Rockaway.

My partner and I responded to a job at a nursing home on the west side of upper Manhattan. A nurse led us down a hallway. As we inquired about the patient's condition, she stated it was one of her co-workers. Upon entering a room, we pushed past the six nurses in a semicircle providing the 'Stare of Care,' I guess they received their training from the FDNY, where firefighters take an advanced course developed for them called, 'The Ring of Concern.'

We found a nurse, approximately forty years old lying on the floor. Her white blouse had been removed and placed *neatly* under her head for comfort. A large, green oxygen tank stood next to her. The only sound was the hiss of the oxygen, blowing like a storm through the attached tubing. At the end of the tubing was a nasal canula (two little prongs that fit in the nose) attached to her nose. I reached over and shut the oxygen off. It did nothing but blow the dust around on the floor. It wasn't doing her any good, she was dead. The nursing staff never recognized that she had suffered a heart attack. Don't even ask about the third world urchin they had for a doctor.

Another time, we were led by a nurse to find an elderly patient on the floor. Her friends sitting holding her hands and wiping her face. We started the Dance of Life, but this person's spirit had departed a while ago and wasn't coming back.

Later, as we consoled the elderly friends, the full story came out. The patient complained about an inability to breathe. The nurse felt she was "acting up" and would be fine after friends gave her some water. Her lungs were already filling with water; and one woman remarked about "those bubbles coming from her mouth."

As the heart attack got worse, the patient started running around the TV room. Her friends pleaded with the nurse to call 911. The nurse consented, only if her friends would "keep her calm." The little old ladies did as they were told. They decided the best move would be to lay their "acting up" friend down.

"She got even more upset," one reported. "But after all of us held her down for a while, she became very calm and went to sleep. Just like the nurse said she would." The old ladies believed their actions helped.

Neither of us had the heart to tell them that by holding her down, they basically assisted in drowning. But then again they did assist her making the transfer to the other side.

Nursing homes were not the only horrors we visited. At the top of the list were doctors' offices. Paramedic Tom Reynolds and I responded to an "inferior wall MI," a deadly heart attack. We pulled up in front of the cardiologist's office north of New York University Hospital in Manhattan.

Entering the office, we were told, "Wait till I get the doctor." The doctor, who worked at NYU, walked in.

"Where's the patient, doctor?" I asked.

"In the waiting room," he responded, pointing the way. Seated among other patients was living death. As we loaded him onto the stretcher, we started the Dance of Life, administering the oxygen, taking the blood pressure, listening to lung sounds, and reading the monitor.

As we worked, the doctor shouted, "I want him in the hospital now."

We both ignored him, until he said those magic words, "I'm ordering you." That did it.

"Exactly what have you done for this patient, doctor?" I asked indignantly.

"Did you give him oxygen? Or perhaps even an aspirin? I won't even ask about nitroglycerin. So what did you do?" I demanded.

"I, uh, called you."

"Fine. We are the paramedics. And unlike you, we are helping the patient."

Then he said in a contrite voice, "Well, I want to be on the team."

"Fine. Get your nurse to make us copies of his record, and you, hold the IV bag, as I start the line."

We transported the patient to NYU, where Doctor Gang from Bellevue began her magic.

Common sense would lead to the conclusion: If you are a cardiologist, or any doctor for that matter, sick people will seek you out. These sick people may crash in front of you and need care. The prudent and sensible thing would be to have the basic medications and instruments for these patients. It seems most doctors are too concerned with the patient's insurance than with the patient and once again *it's all about the money.*

Then there were the *Clinics* and the 'cab rides' to their affiliated hospitals.

They always put in a call to 911 for a ride to the hospital. It was their policy whether the person had a stubbed toe or had an asthma attack, the clinics strained the 911 system with transport jobs that were, for the most part, unnecessary. Had the union the vision, they could have connected MetroCare or American Medical Response to cover these jobs, keeping 911 units free to do emergencies. It would have also relieved some of the strain FDEMS units were already under. But the union, as the chiefs, were playing the fear factor, continuously reminding us these other organizations were after our jobs. The result was self-promoting and denying the public a better-developed resource.

The usual was the "difficulty breathing" six-year-old, with an asthma history. It just so happened the clinic was closing, so they called 911.

They sometimes loaded the kids up with Albuterol, but did nothing to educate the family, or provide antibiotics for the underlying infection that precipitated the attack.

A doctor at the San Juan Clinic called us about a woman who weighed more than 400 pounds and had "slight CHF" (congestive heart failure). When Angelo Morales and I got this oversized heifer into the back of the bus, we started our evaluation. She was in third-degree heart block! In this condition, the top of the heart, the atria, didn't know what the bottom of the heart, the ventricles, were doing. They marched to different beats, similar to the Street Saints of Compassion and the civilian chiefs, or doctors in these Bodega Clinics of medicine. The tune being played was "Knock, Knock, Knocking on Heaven's Door." We worked getting her into the hospital, alive, no thanks to the buffoon 'Doc in the box' at San Juan Clinic.

South Bronx patients, to reiterate, are likely to be of a minority, so who gave a shit? The EMS crews who saw these patients every day, that's who. *We gave a shit.*

Here is another example of how the Mayor protected his own, thus answering the question why the Gestapo (BITS) didn't go after the MetroCare crew that had a child in cardiac arrest, but drove to Presbyterian Medical Center (a private hospital) in Manhattan, passing Lincoln (a City)

Hospital in the South Bronx. Nothing happened to 'Rudy's EMS.'

It's interesting to note history in the fact that Giuliani attempted to destroy Health and Hospitals by wiping out the 911 Committee, allowing for no checks and balances as to the care people, especially minorities, received.

I also find it interesting that he has always been known as a micromanager and that before him there was Ed Koch. The significance here is that his father, before being admitted to Sing Sing Prison, underwent a psychiatric exam by the then City's Department of Hospitals. Having a background in Forensic Psychology from John Jay College of Criminal Justice, I find it extremely interesting to note what Psychiatrist Benjamin Apfelberg wrote to Judge Bohan of the evaluation. "A study of these individuals makeup reveals that he is a personality deviate of the aggressive, egocentric type. He is egocentric to an extent where <u>he has failed to consider the feelings and rights of others."</u>

Oh, concerning former Mayor Koch, Mr. Giuliani Senior, worked for Koch Plumbing for only two weeks. His crime, by the way was robbery with a weapon.

For my own part after seeing his son, our mayor, at work, especially with minorities, that old saying "Like father, like son" rang true for me. Is there a vindictive connection especially between his glee to destroy Health and Hospitals and the report issued about his father by the City's Department of Health? I certainly don't know, but . . . And yet, unlike his father who was more brawn than brains, I could clearly see the now-mayor had realized that he could never match his father's physical prowess. What I saw was him crafting his skills of intimidation, becoming a master of attacking people ad hominem: playing on emotions <u>instead of facts</u>, and <u>*on fears instead of truths*</u>.

Like him or not, one had to respect his arrogant tenacity and never underestimate his formable base of financial and emotional support.

This, in my opinion, was where the leadership of Local 2507 totally failed in their perception of the threat.

Concerning his and Governor Pataki's buddy, Steve Zakheim? If you'd like to learn more concerning Governor Pataki and nursing homes, please investigate and you'll see how he rewarded his contributors. Some things never change. Headlines of an article in the November 29, 2003 New York Post would report yet another story that the gentlemen "participated in a scheme to defraud Medicare of $34 million, according to federal authorities." Like I said, the fruit doesn't fall far from the tree and I'm not talking about the former mayor's cross-dressing sessions while doing a show. But I would like to know how a convicted felon has a 'carry' weapon permit in NYC?

Here is an incident kept from the public by the EMS chiefs after it was learned the micromanaging, egocentric mayor screwed up. A kid met the trauma criteria and needed to go to a trauma center. The mother wanted to go to Presbyterian, which was neither a trauma center *nor* close. Her husband was "a doctor" there. Giuliani, newly elected mayor, ordered the EMS lieutenant to have the child taken to Presbyterian. The officer conscious of the political repercussions followed the directive as did the crew.

The child suffered the extra distance and then had to be removed to a trauma center, where the EMS crew was originally headed.

Needless to say nothing was said in regards to the new mayor putting his nose where it should have never been or demanding and intimidating an EMS officer and crew to get another cash cow donating doctor on his bandwagon.

While Chief of EMS Command Robert McCracken and Assistant Commissioner for Emergency Medicine John J. Clair vigorously defended MetroCare and its president, Steve Zakheim, to the city council and local community boards, patient trust was violated. The city council and local community boards, including mayoral hopefuls like Council

Speaker Peter Vallone, should have listened and vigorously inquired about McCracken's rumored "Special Supervisor" position in MetroCare. Whether the rumor was true or not again common sense would have dictated a closer look, yet it never happened.

To reiterate, this was another opportunity for Local 2507 to make its point, but by this time they were now waging yet another losing battle over the FD allowing New York Cornell and other "voluntary" hospitals to place extra units on the street. Once again, in my humble opinion, there were more pressing emergent problems. The paramedics and EMTs of NY Cornell are some of the most knowledgeable and professional in the country. Who can argue with the likes of paramedics Andy Margolies, Steve Friend, or Lori Beninson? The lesson here is division is unnatural. Unity and the acceptance of diversity can only enrich patient care.

The union also failed to capitalize on the plight of Lincoln Hospital a City Hospital understaffing, overworked staff and the negative impact it was having on the community thanks to the mayor. It had a dedicated emergency room staff that gave us a good run for the money when we were in trouble with a patient. They were the best I'd seen in the South Bronx concerning trauma, at the time. Another great facility was Albert Einstein Hospital, which always tried to do right by the patient, having the most professional nursing staff in the Bronx.

On August 1, 2001, EMS Command Order 2001-039 was issued. It stated: "The New York State Department of Health has designated (Hospital #83) Saint Barnabas Hospital as a regional trauma center in New York City."

Working out of Battalion Twenty-six, I had the pleasure to meet and work with doctor Juan Acosta (D.O.), a former paramedic. He worked with the EMS crews and took suggestions to the administrators at Saint Barnabas. Because of his dedication to patient care, and follow-up, the facility finally changed for the positive in less than six months. Yes, Dr. Juan Acosta pushed hard to give the community better health care. But would you expect less from someone who is, and always will be, a street paramedic at heart? He was the connection between the book-learned pundits of medicine and a well-balanced healer. Although Barnabas was still light years behind Bellevue, it was my choice when I got sick and had to be transported to the hospital. I owe the staff heartfelt thanks and believe that good things will happen if the administration will continue to not only listen but _hear_ what the doctor is saying.

Five
The Implosion Continued

Juan Acosta as well as the administrators at St. Barnabas understood Paulo Freire's statement that "authentic thinking, that is concerned about reality, does not take place in ivory tower isolation, but only in communication" (Pedagogy of the Oppressed, p. 77). If that didn't suit your taste, it should be noted that former Clinton administration Treasury Secretary Robert Rubin, in his book 'In an Uncertain World', espoused the necessity of being open to experiences and opinions as well as the importance of respecting individual dignity. Sadly, within FDNY EMS this was not the case. As time went on, the pressure increasingly fell upon the shoulders of the EMTs and paramedics as the chiefs, cowering to their taskmaster, the FDNY commissioner, sought to distance themselves from the people working the streets.

Not one of them ever read Freire's work yet they had lived up to his model concerning oppressors. The world they developed portrayed them as men, in their own minds. "But for them, to be men is to be oppressors. This is their model of humanity. This phenomenon derives from the fact that the oppressed at a certain moment of their existential experience, adopt an attitude of 'adhesion' to the oppressor." (p. 45) Thus in the end, as the adhesion with the whims of the fire com-missioner gelled, any chance of self-identity as intellectual thinkers evaporated. EMS chiefs reflected the belief that "the oppressor, who himself is dehumanized because he dehumanizes others . . . cannot love because they love only themselves" (p. 55). Loving and caring for themselves, they focused on their own survival and self-inflated the shallow shadows of the men and women they could have been. Thus the paperwork and charges for minor infractions increased as they attempted to get blood from stones.

Battalion Twenty-six was located at east One Hundred Sixty-ninth Street and Boston Road. The sound of R&B, rap, and Spanish music filled the air. In a lot of ways, the burned-out building across the street, undergoing rehab, reminded me of Bosnia during the war. The block included the Soap Opera Laundromat, Asona African Restaurant, and Sing Sing Chinese Restaurant. The Alive Chapel International, with Pastor Elisa Salife Amoako, was directly across the street.

Next door were a barbershop and a car wash. All were establishments of hardworking people. The streets were choked with the double- and triple-parked cars and ambulances. Some of the crews had been parking the ambulances in the bus stop across the way. Someone called in a complaint, so a dictate was sent down from Puzzle Palace (Headquarters at Nine Metro Tech)—Operating Guide Revision Notice 113-03 dated May 3, 2000—and sent to the field on November 20, 2000.

It stated in part, "This is to notify all personnel that, effective immediately, they will be held strictly accountable for the timely disposition of parking summons issued to department vehicles in their use. Such violations include, but are not limited to, 'No Standing,' 'No Parking,' 'Double Parking,' 'Fire Hydrants'." Thus, if DOT (Department of Traffic) ticketed ambulances, the crew paid.

I didn't see this happening to the heroes in their little red trucks (firefighters). They had a long history of abusing their power. Hell, they'd even killed a person going to a Chinese restaurant for dinner in Queens with lights and sirens. Then they physically kept the medics from getting to the injured person, who later died.

EMS Administration, in those early days before the merger, remained true to form. In a press interview, they tried, in vain, to blame the EMS crew for insubordination and cover up the Bravest's deed. They said they lost the ACR and the radio tapes making Richard Nixon's story almost plausible. In the end, the street-smart crew turned the tables on supervision and administration. They went to the press, as well as to the court, with a copy of the ACR. Soon after, crews were told it was illegal to make copies of ACRs. That ruling remains. Some things never change.

Paramedic Angelo Morales, and I sat in Twenty-six William. It was a typical day in the barrio. A Spanish male came up to the unit, attempting to hand me a bottle of water. I graciously refused, but we both agreeably accepted after my partner spoke to him in Spanish.

The man had suffered a heart attack and was unconscious when an EMS unit got to him. They worked him and later he left the hospital. He never learned the names of the crew members. Yet, unlike so many others we serve, he didn't forget.

Angelo explained he had heard of the man we had just met. He would come out of his shop when a bus was parked in front and give the crew bottled water, hoping in some small way to thank the crew members who saved his life. The Street Saints of Compassion, the unknown crew, left an indelible mark.

A female medic in a Bronx Battalion had gone on a job with her partner. The patient was HIV positive. He was speaking to her as she worked on him. As he spoke, he unintentionally spit and she was hit in her eye. After treating and transporting the patient to the hospital, she went back to the Battalion and reported it to her supervisor. He had her fill out an Exposure Form. Once it was complete, he ordered the crew to go back to available status.

At the very least, she expected the supervisor to say that he was sorry for what happened, or for him to reach out in some type of compassionate manner. Instead, he was more concerned about putting the unit back into service.

Three days later, BHS called, saying the patient was HIV positive. The medic *should have immediately* gone to the emergency room to start the "cocktail" of medications use for AIDS exposure.

She went out on LODI (line of duty injuries make her unable to continue her job), but lost precious time. The supervisor was only interested in keeping a unit available, not in the silent death sentence given to a member of his command.

EMS Supervision will never allow FDNY to outdo them in pushing the envelope of stupidity. Lt. Paul Giblin could never hold a candle to these three you are about to read about. One night, a medic unit was pulling out of Bellevue EMS Station Thirteen. The driver couldn't go forward because the yard was blocked. The supervisor, Lt. Rob Russo (nicknamed Carrot Top for his red flaming hair), had failed to keep the yard open, thus the paramedic had to back up. As he was backing out, he heard a scream and stopped.

The screaming stopped, so he backed up, but again the scream.

"Where the hell is it coming from?"

"I don't know. It's a woman's voice," said the partner, both exhausted from the lack of air conditioning in the front of the unit, combined with working mandatory overtime shifts EMS management could not fill because they failed to hire enough people. The combination could prove lethal and almost did. Thus it was either work overtime or face losing a day's pay.

As they started to back out the third time, a woman frantically screamed. The crew stopped and looked around. The screams came from a nursing student, across the street. She pointed to the back of the bus. The driver opened his door, looked back, and saw two feet.

Moving the bus forward they jumped out. Under the rear wheels of the bus was a homeless drunk with multiple leg fractures and a fractured pelvis. The crew grabbed the equipment, stabilized the patient, packaging the patient while notifying the dispatcher then took him to the nearest trauma center. The nearest trauma center was Bellevue Hospital and since the EMS garage was on Bellevue grounds, it took perhaps four minutes.

The crew members did the right thing for the patient. However, the idiot supervisor wanted the crew members brought up on charges for "leaving the scene of an accident and tampering with evidence."

Nothing was done to help the traumatized crew. ISU showed up to do a urine sample, but nothing was done to help the crew members. Instead, the anal lieutenant sought charges against them.

Do you still wonder why EMS supervisors are so loved? Their statements have literally killed people. By the way, no charges were ever brought against the inept clown behind the desk who created the hazardous condition in the first place. If the crew members were guilty it was for not having a member walk behind the rear of the bus.

Another classic sign of a leader is one who is alert to all that is happening around him. One such leader was Lieutenant Richard Cooper. Richie had a medical problem that played havoc with his eyesight.

Paramedic Adam Brynes and I were turning in the drugs at the end of a tour when Lieutenant Cooper went ballistic. He emptied the room of everyone except us.

I flipped the drugs to Adam who was about to place them in the security locker when he was told, "Stop! I want to see your drugs."

We both looked at each other then the lieutenant who was an EMT, not a paramedic. Point being he wouldn't know morphine from ice cream. But we complied.

"You don't take this seriously, do you, Schrang?" he snapped. He reached in the desk drawer and proceeded to kneel in front of the drugs. Next he measured each one.

Our tour was over; we were not getting paid overtime. Yet we were being royally abused. Adam tried to give him a hint, but he wouldn't take it.

As he went to recheck the drugs a second time, I looked at him and said, "You're an asshole." This got his attention and caused a bit of a ruckus, but we finally got the drugs locked up and left.

Another night, someone played a videotape on the large-screen TV in the lounge, of two homosexuals. It was brought to the good lieutenant's attention so he ran into the lounge and knelt in front of the TV to inspect. As one male received a blow-job, Richie's head bobbed back and forth, yes gentle reader it looked like you just read it. The only thing missing was a camera at this point. His eyesight was so bad he had difficulty finding the switch for the VCR. When he realized the VCR was beyond his technical capability, he got off his knees and ran upstairs to the captain. "Captain! Two men are doing it in the lounge."

Needless to say, the captain and the lieutenant never figured out who did this dastardly deed. They even went so far as to inquire at the local video store.

I want all you badass sons and daughter's of a camel flea's shit (Al Qaeda assholes) to pay attention, your rat infested training camps will never give you training like this. Put the bombs, chemicals, and nukes away and watch how one idiot can crash the world's largest system with might I add… one finger! Your gutless leader can't do this.

Lieutenant Richard Cooper was nicknamed the "Computer Whiz." One night the good lieutenant was sending out a message to all boroughs for an ALS (paramedic) vacancy. Somehow, the 'send' button was locked into place. Talk about a single man crashing the system. More than three hundred messages were sent! At the same time, the phone to the office wasn't working.

When it rains it pours in the delusional EMS kingdom of ineptness. Chief McCracken the chief of the world's largest EMS watched his world melting down. The only solution this genius came up with was to make a less than polite phone call to Captain Stone, Lt. Cooper's boss at home in Long Island! The captain and the chief were already on endearing terms, since the chief had gone after the captain's unauthorized 'gator' hat.

They could not even notify the lieutenant by radio, because he didn't have one! Finally, a patrol boss took it upon himself to drive back to the garage and literally pull the plug on the machine!

Another lieutenant at a station had a problem with alcohol. The guy had a legitimate medical problem. He was on numerous stipulations, and though he violated them, they continually brought him back to work after he dried out. This would seem like a fair deal, except I had not seen it evenly administered when it came to the medics and EMTs. He was also the first to write people up for being a few minutes late or for taking too many of their earned sick days while he was AWOL (absent without leave) on a binge.

One day, there was an MVA. A Basic unit along with Paramedic Tommy Reynolds and I were dispatched. When we got there, people were trying to decide whether to go to the hospital or not. It was basically a fender bender they were out of the vehicles and sitting, some standing on the sidewalk. Once again, the EMT's, who do the majority of the work, did the right thing.

The patrol boss pulled up just as the EMT's convinced the people to go to the hospital to be checked, instead of walking off the scene. Right away, the lieutenant got into the black EMT's face. He wanted to know why these people weren't stabilized and taken from the car. I broke it up because it was spiraling toward the 'boss' getting his ass kicked, the EMT going to jail, and the patients not getting appropriate care.

After arriving at the ER I told the crew to remain inside until I came for them. I walked outside to the agitated lieutenant and got in the command car. The lieutenant made it clear that operating procedures had not been followed.

"That EMT was a wise ass and I have to do the paperwork and write him up."

The lieutenant usually worked a different shift and did not know this crew; we did. We worked with them every day and they were great. Besides once you work the streets long enough you can tell when there is a racial undercurrent and it had been detected by both by me and EMT. I explained that the EMT's arrived after the people were ambulatory and wanted to leave the scene. It was them out of caring for the people that convinced them to be seen at the hospital.

The EMT in question was waiting to go to the fire side to become a firefighter and would not be allowed if he had charges pending against him. Since the lieutenant appeared to relish the idea of destroying the kid's future confirming my racial hunch, I decided to take another route. Pretending to smelled something and I went for the throat.

"Sir, I see you are determined to write the crew up, but may I ask you a question off the record?"

"Sure, we've known each other for years."

"Great. Then you know I'm very concerned about you and, well, your breath. Have you been drinking again?"

"What? Oh, no. It's my mouthwash!"

"Okay, if you say so. But I'm really worried about you and it is certainly not your mouthwash. I was just wondering."

"Smell my cologne."

"That's okay. If you tell me you are clean, I'm glad. By the way concerning the crew . . ." Before I could finish, he blurted out, "Tell them to go back into service. There will be no paperwork."

"Cool. See you later, boss and I'd suggest a different mouthwash."

I told the crew to avoid saying anything to him and got in my unit. I told Tommy what transpired and he laughed hysterically. Then he looked at me saying, "When will they ever learn?" The good lieutenant disappeared and didn't show up for another two weeks. The EMT did go to fire department. Years later the officer remarried and cleaned up his act totally, thus the reason I've not listed his name.

After being sent to the Bronx I was back under Civilian Deputy Chief Villani's command. I knew it was just a matter of time before he got to me. I wasn't feeling very chipper after hearing that paramedic Richard Stein died on December 19, 2000, reportedly from Hepatitis C. Rich was one of three New York City paramedics who went with me to Bosnia during the genocide. He was a great guy. I was in no mood for EMS administrative bullshit, but when it rains it pours in EMS land. However just like the rain one had to measure the stupidity to really get a feel for it.

The first issue came up when Captain Mittleman, never known for other than being a "Yes man" and as far as I was concerned a self serving back stabber showed me a note from Villani stating he wanted a copy of my DD 214 (discharge from the military). When I showed the captain my pension check from the Veteran's Administration, it would be months before I would receive my DD 214, he asked,

"Why are you busting my balls? That's not good enough." I guess the Veteran's Administration gives checks out to anyone now, but that gentle reader was only the first drop.

On Christmas Eve, 2000, the good captain gave me a shopping list from Villani. It was a list of "multiple performance issues."

Ok, now we are into the storm. The Christmas list went as follows:

High activation times." (It took me a minute and seventeen seconds to press the 10-63 button on the computer. It usually took longer than that for the job to appear on the computer screen.)

"No 10-81 signal." (I was at the hospital, but should have been more concerned about if my signal went through, than getting the patient into the emergency room.)

High travel time." (We were a South Bronx paramedic unit, but had to cover other areas. In this case, he inquired about a twenty-three-minute response time. On the day I received this, we did one job outside our battalion and division that took forty minutes travel time, including getting lost.)

"Inappropriate mileage entry." (The KDT, onboard computer system, left much to be desired. I always put in 99999 as a mileage and never had a problem logging on. Captain Mittleman told me he wanted this corrected.

However when the exact mileage went in, the computer kicked it back, "inappropriate mileage." I asked him to witness it, but instead he sent an EMT to confirm it under the plausible denial defense concept. Better than twenty minutes into the tour, I finally got logged on, doing what I was ordered to do. The next day the same problem occurred. This time, a lieutenant witnessed it.)

"Out of service on 10-100 Emergency at Battalion Twenty-six, twelve minutes prior to the end of tour after spending one hour 10-81."(If Villani had read the sheet correctly, he'd have noticed that, from 16:30 hours till 17:48 hours, we were in our unit. That's one hour and eighteen minutes sitting in the unit.

The bottom line was that EMS communication had stated there would be no breaks, bathroom or not, in the last hour. All the crews felt the same. When you have to go, you go... Besides, the officer at the desk saw me in the bathroom.

It was Christmas Eve and I'd received a shopping list to answer. The captain got his answers in a seven-page document the day after Christmas.

The paperwork answered all the questions *and offered suggestions.*

For my effort, Captain Mittleman told me, "It was entertaining, but people will think you're a wise guy. Chief Villani does not want solutions, just answers." I could understand this coming from a guy who couldn't come up with a solution to save his life after being an ass wipe paper pushing "Yes" man all his life. Talk about oxymoron, or in this case just morons.

As he spoke, my mind drifted off to a tune playing on the TV in the office. It was the Beatles singing the hit, "Nowhere Man." I tried not to laugh, as I heard the words, "Making all his plans for nobody." That's what this wannabee civilian EMS DC, like the rest, was doing. I turned back to the captain as he spoke.

"You make reference to his (Villani) giving a CD to a paramedic for getting into an accident, by responding lights and sirens to a call. You tie this in with BITS filming a crew sitting in traffic with lights on, using due regard. Both have *nothing to do with you*."

Indeed it did. The paramedic got the CD after she did paperwork for an EEO, because she felt threatened by the civilian deputy chief. Thus he ordered a certain captain, guess who to write the CD.

If he wanted my response time to improve and I pushed the envelope, I could expect to pay out of my pocket. I think not. The *problem* was in the appropriate utilization of resources. To cover his ass, he punished those who tried, instead of correcting the problem. This was nothing new with Civilian DC Villani.

As I stood there Captain Mittleman reiterated, "He doesn't want solutions."

I rewrote the package and included this quote from Dante, "Abandon hope, all ye who enter here." Oh and by the way, Captain Mittleman became a Deputy Chief; are we noting a pattern here or is it just me?

My partner Angelo Morales told me of being mandated **for wearing sunglasses**. On this occasion an officer from ISU (Inspectional Services Unit) was out stalking units as usual. As the crew sat trying to relax in the cramped cab, listening to the radio, the officer approached with stealth. Angelo caught the officer next to his window. Rolling it down, he was informed in a belligerent manner, "Report back to your station!"

Once back, the desk supervisor yelled at him for "sleeping" and produced his "evidence." It was a Polaroid photo this supervisor had taken. It showed the crew member sitting up wearing sunglasses. This is the same "officer" that was caught in Manhattan breaking into a car, in uniform, by the police! Seems if you needed a part, this was the man who, when not reportedly doing 'white snow' (cocaine) he was heisting parts off cars. This day the car he was attempting to rip off belonged to an injured fireman who had called the precinct, requesting that the sector drive by just to check his car till he was able to pick it up. Lo and behold, as the sector pulled up, there was an EMS Command vehicle next to the car in question. The hood was up and our hapless officer was working on removing a carburetor.

When questioned, he claimed it was his vehicle at which time the cops brought him in. Nothing ever came of this because the officer was married to a very-high-ranking woman of position in Health and Hospitals.

On 9-11-'01 'shit head' was found sitting on a sidewalk, crying hysterically, of no value in assisting EMS crew members save patients.

Captain Mark Stone pulled a similar fiasco with my unit, and a basic unit sitting in front of us. I was the one wearing the sunglasses. As the KDT went off, I checked it and went back to napping. My partner Arty was on his cell phone, talking long distance to his mother. Standing on my partner's side, the captain banged on the window scarring the hell out of Arty who yelled and at the same time was disconnected from Mom in Puerto Rico.

"You both could have been killed if I had a gun!" he yelled. "Get off that cell phone. It's unauthorized!"

"Fuck off. Get a life, will you!" I said as Arty, now furious muttered how the captain upset his mother, who was left thinking something happened since he cut the conversation.

Unrelenting, the captain headed for the basic unit parked in front of us. I jumped out and banged the window of the crew member in the front, waking him up.

"Where's your partner? I caught you sleeping," the captain joyously proclaimed proceeding to the back door banging on it. It opened and the EMT got out.

"How was your sleep?" the captain asked, gloating over his prize.

"Fine," said the EMT wearing a T-shirt, not a uniform shirt.

"Get to your street corner, now."

Captain Mark Stone could not wait to get back to Bellevue to tell everyone he caught crews sleeping and have the lieutenant write them up. The crew in question did a lot of overtime covering slots for these officers. In the end, both workers quit EMS, two more EMS success stories while Captain Mark Stone nicknamed "Lollipop" in the South Bronx waited to be a deputy chief.

I was outside an office when I heard one supervisor at Battalion Twenty-six get a call from another supervisor. It seemed the patrol boss had found the crew members sleeping and was asking the desk officer what to do. The patrol boss was on overtime and not from that battalion. The supervisor on the desk said, "They worked the midnight tour and volunteered to work this shift. Do whatever you want."

Neither incident was anything but typical EMS harassment. If the captain or the supervisor had an ounce of brains, they would have asked the dispatcher to contact the unit. If they did not answer, then give them a tone. Failing that put them out of service. _Then it would be justified._

Short of that, it was self-serving, egomania. Our people did not need this and deserved better.

Paul Giblin, Navy Seal Wannabe, and I must have been brothers in a former life. I say this because I kept hoping against hope, that one day he would stand by his people and demonstrate leadership. He had no idea how many times I literally saved his life.

One warm afternoon at Bellevue I noted several EMTs standing by the fence under the shade of the tree.

What really caught my attention were their eyes. Each pair followed the Navy Seal as he exited his car and waddled toward the bathroom for his pre-tour HAZMAT (Hazardous Material)strike. Approaching, I heard them discussing placing clear cellophane on the toilet seat and coating it with nitro paste. The nitro would have bottomed his blood pressure, rendering him unconscious on the cellophane.

I pointed out that ESU of the police department would have to be called to remove the door, come to think of it, part of the wall also to get to the unconscious Seal. Besides, who would want to witness such a sight? He would be deep in his own shit, and, even more importantly, who would go into that toxic environment to work him? Just the thought was enough to curdle milk and frayed their nerves enough to realize it wasn't an option.

So the crew settled on going up to New York Hospital with a mannequin. They strapped it to a plastic long board, placed a sign on it reading:

"Navy Seal Paul Giblin, Help!" and launched it into the river to release some stress of another night of having Paul Giblin Navy Seal on patrol.

Another time, an irate EMT was going to lace his drink with an LSD tablet he'd taken off an overdosed patient. Although instrumental in saving the Seal from a certain trip to the quiet room in the Bellevue Psychiatry Department, I must admit it would have been cool to witness. Even I was getting pushed more than my good nature could accept.

Debbie Smith, another fun partner and good paramedic, told me a story that happened when she was an EMT. She and another female partner responded to a "suicidal EDP." When they got to the scene, they found the man locked in his bathroom, threatening to kill himself. They called for the police and a patrol boss.

While waiting for the resources to arrive, the EMTs talked the suicidal male out of the bathroom into the living room. He left the bathroom, knife in hand, still threatening to kill himself, and to hurt them.

The girls were determined. Without backup, these true Street Saints of Compassion remained with the armed man. They valued his life more than he did. Through their compassionate approach, they got the man to surrender his knife.

The EMS patrol boss finally showed up. As he was assessing the situation, the EMT gave the weapon to the boss. The suicidal man asked the lieutenant for the weapon and the lieutenant *gave it back to him*. To top it off, the lieutenant, who was a paramedic, wanted the crew to let the patient sign the ACR so they could leave.

The crew decided to call telemetry. As Debbie talked to a doctor, her partner got the weapon away from the man for a second time. Hearing the situation, the doctor tore into Debbie until she told him the order was from the lieutenant on the scene.

"Put him on the phone, now!"

Needless to say, the EDP was brought to the hospital, and the other EDP (the lieutenant) went back on patrol. The lieutenant continued to lead a confused life and was transferred from one station to another. Even though he'd violated the integrity of a double-keyed, narcotic locker on another occasion, the idiot remained a lieutenant, yes, only the best for EMS. Would you expect less?

One call type we receive a lot was "unknown condition" calls. Commonsense would dictate the police should be dispatched first. Then if a bus was needed, send the appropriate call type. But who were we to question the Communication Division?

If they want a better system, make the dispatchers civilians. Who the hell needs an EMT to dispatch? Often we get a subway job and the computer displays, **"Fire assigned. Fire closed. Unable to validate address."**

In the above case, an engine company was assigned. But they closed the job. Why? **"Unable to validate**

address." If there was no smoke to smell or flames to see, or cameras present for a photo opt, then and only then could the Bravest find the job.

Think we were not prepared leading up to 9-11-01? One day at Battalion Eight, Bellevue, Lt. Paul Giblin, Navy Seal, was in charge, sitting behind the desk. An EMT reported to the good lieutenant that there was a "strange briefcase" on the wooden bench outside his office. Not being one to miss a threat, Paul Giblin, Navy Seal, called in a "suspicious package." ESU came, followed by fire department and our useless chiefs, SOD (Special Operations Division), the Bomb Squad.

The hospital administrator was contemplating an evacuation. Everybody was suited up, awaiting the mobile bomb rover to pick up the suspicious package when EMT Reggie Jenkins walked in from the cafeteria. Everyone yelled as he went over and recovered *his briefcase*. You can't put anything over on EMS supervision.

Talking about being on top of things, Lieutenant Correa from Battalion Twenty-six went to great lengths to inform me that Chief Gumbo had asked for his advice concerning making up a lieutenant's exam. As he expounded on the job of being a boss, paramedic Debbie Smith stood behind him, listening. Later she told me the following story concerning his knowledge of the job.

Just finished working her unit she decided to work overtime on a BLS unit with an EMT. The EMTs are issued, let's say, only four Albuterol treatments per oxygen bag. Albuterol is placed in a nebulizer and administered to a patient with asthma. A medic has unlimited access to the treatment since we carry extras in our oxygen bag, as well as our primary drug bag.

Lieutenant Correa saw Debbie place some extra Albuterol in her pocket and yelled, "That's ALS (paramedic) Albuterol. It's a different dosage from BLS (EMT) Albuterol."

It's all the same, gentle reader but he didn't know it. Yet this was the same individual who completed our evaluation sheets. Even if he showed up on the scene, how could he judge what my partner or I were doing, when he was an EMT and not a paramedic? Yet an EMS chief asked him to prepare an exam. Does it surprise you?

Navy Seal wannabe, Lieutenant Paul Giblin, was transferred to Metropolitan Hospital Battalion Ten after he tried to use his imagined authority on one of the staff from the ridiculous television program Third Watch, who was filming at Bellevue.

Captain Stone quickly signed his transfer.

The next time I saw Paul, Paramedic Angelo Morales and I brought a patient into Mount Sinai Hospital in Manhattan. I introduced him to Angelo and he explained how Captain Phil Para,(No Neck) had made him executive officer. I smiled and wished him well.

"What a ship of fools that place must be," I remarked to Angelo.

"So that's the Navy Seal, huh?" he asked, with an understanding grin.

A rather remarkable thing happened one night in February concerning Civilian DC Villani. Angelo and I pulled up in Twenty-six William and saw him standing by the garage entrance. As I got out of the unit and retrieved my gear, he approached.

"It's taken me a while to hook up with you, Schrang. Good evening."

He extended his hand, so I shook it. "I hear from the captain that you are getting comfortable up here. He has no complaints."

"Well, I have two great partners and love working in this shithole helping people. The hospital care is a joke. Listen, are you done with the bullshit?" I asked, as people gathered by the office to listen to what was transpiring.

"What do you mean?" he asked soberly.

"I mean, you tried to get me fired over a bullshit CCU report that had nothing to do with me. In fact, the doctor said I did a fantastic job. The complaint was about my partner and her big mouth.

Next, you tried to get me to pay for equipment. McCracken overruled the judgment, and once again you had egg on your face. Just what the fuck did I ever do to you?"

"That was a different borough," he said.

"What's this crap with sending a list, asking why our response time is so long, or why it's taking a minute and so many seconds to hit the damn button?"

"Oh, I don't remember that," he responded.

"I hear you chiefs are hanging on by a thread. Did you know anything about changing your title to 'unit managers' so the fire battalion chiefs can take over when they get rid of you?" I asked.

"No. Basile (Division Commander, EMS Division Five, known as The Snake) said we beat fire in court."

"I sure hope so but I wouldn't believe too much The Snake (Basile) has to say. But to be perfectly honest, you know the chiefs have always *been the problem* from the days of Becker. I was hoping you would all be fired up, once we were given as sacrificial lambs to fire. I was hoping for adult leadership for a change."

He stood there, silently listening.

"You guys, each of you chiefs had your moment in history to grow a pair of balls at the merger. If you had a pair, or even backbone, and had the leadership ability we now have in Pat Bahnken (Union President), it would have been a different world. It was the EMTs and medics that made this merger work. Not fire."

"You are right," he said. Then he made a statement that startled me.

"At the merger, fire told us we were not needed. I could not afford to take a thirty-thousand-dollar-a-year cut."

"Well," I said softly, "if my back is against the wall and you are telling me I will lose everything on your whim, then I will take you down, going balls to the wall. This is what you guys should have done."

"I know," he replied.

"Concerning my reassignment here, do you know what happened?" I asked.

"I heard you had an argument with someone."

"No, *I followed orders*," I said.

"Well, that will always get you in trouble," he said, reflecting on a thought.

I explained the situation to him finishing by telling him about the Federal EEO charges I had placed. I looked straight into his tired eyes.

"Between Stone and Iannarelli neither wanted to act like adults in addressing the problem of Grillo. So what they feared, an EEO, bit each of them in the ass. Fuck with me, and I have nothing to lose. I go federal."

We said our goodnights. I walked toward my partner and others who were waiting to hear what happened.

"What did he say?" they asked.

"Oh, Villani, he's now my buddy." They really looked surprised. Then I added, "Remember the old Chinese saying: 'Keep your friends close. Your enemy much closer."

I smiled as they bowed honorably. I'm not known as "Old Ancient Wise One" for nothing.

I waited to see how long it would take for the captain to approach me, to see how the meeting went. I'm sure Villani wanted to know. As I expected, he approached and hung around until being told of the 'talk'. I told him I was pleased, and I honestly was, that we spoke.

So long as there was two-way conversation, there wouldn't be guessing, miscalculations, or fear. I didn't trust him, but I felt good that we spoke.

I hoped this would end the bullshit he had with me. But time and deeds would tell, not words. I was pleased he admitted what I had long preached.

My partner and friend, Angelo Morales, had a joke I modified to include FDNY EMS chiefs.

"What do whores, politicians, and lawyers have in common?"

The answer is, "Give them money and they will take any position."

After DC Villani made his honest statement, I added the chiefs to the joke.

On February 20, 2001, I took the train into the city. It was an overcast day, as I headed toward city hall to join several hundred brothers and sisters supporting President Pat Bahnken as he represented us in a bid to get Uniform Status. This would mean we would no longer be classified as "civilians" and we'd be in position to bargain for ourselves within DC37.

The city representative spoke first. I looked at the overweight, disheveled individual who spoke against us. He popped Certs in a mouth located amidst jowls of fat. No sweets, no matter how strong, could hide the disdain he had for us thinking to myself, this is the same fat slob who will be begging us to save his pencil pushing shit life one day. Looking like he did, it would be in his own best interest to have a highly trained, well-equipped EMS team.

First Deputy Fire Commissioner Feehan sat next to him. The man projected negativity as dark as a bottle of cheap red wine I'm sure he knew well. Hey it's my impression! His words were typical of Fire God tradition, lies.

Within two weeks of the hearing, Peter Gorman the no-nonsense president of the Uniform Fire Officers Association (UFOA) made a public statement of support and testified as such, but nothing is as it appears. He, being a shrewd politician saw an opportunity to bring heat on his boss using us to get what he wanted for *his* firefighters. But even more remarkably he stated, "We have no confidence in Fire Commissioner's (Thomas Von Essen) ability to run this department." Further, regarding the merger, he stated, "We were lied to."

As for the Fire God, Von Essen and his two fire puppets, Fire Department Chief Ganci and First Deputy

117

Commissioner Feehan, Mr. Gorman said, "These egotistical individuals claim to know how to run the world's largest EMS."

First Deputy Commissioner Feehan sat in front of the city council. We heard lies from his mouth concerning our quest for Uniform Status. He reiterated promises the fire department made so the merger would be granted by the city council five years ago.

To his left sat the "poster child" in uniform, EMS Chief Robert McCracken. He had fooled a lot of people, including me through the years claiming to "govern by the people," having come up through the ranks. He thought, as all political ass wipes do that he could delude everyone into believing he was there "for the people."

As I sat in the hallowed chamber of New York City government, I looked up. In the ceiling's rotunda was the statement, "Governed by the people, for the people."

McCracken, like Villani, was no longer of the people of EMS. They sold their souls for a few pieces of gold. To his credit, Villani admitted it.

When asked how much it would cost the city to give us Uniform Status, the fat slob representing the city did not know. When asked about the impact, he did not know.

In reality, it would cost them nothing. Everything would be gained in bargaining. It would make the workforce happy. Herein lay another EMS FD truth. If EMS command, towing the line for the Fire God, could do something, *anything* to benefit the workforce, or make their lives more miserable, they would always opt for the latter with zest.

The city council members led by Walter McCaffrey, Victor Robles, and Ronnie Eldrige saw right through the lies. I was glad I went. The city council did grant us Uniform Status, but the mayor took them to court to block it.

Looking at McCracken with his awards pinned to his chest a song ran through my head which could be applied to him and 99.9 percent of the EMS supervisors, "The Backstabbers" by the OJ's.

Six

Fire Follies

A Proud History of Over 135 Years Unimpeded by Progress
or
Common Sense

The New York City Fire Department was founded in 1865. I stand in total awe at the untiring efforts to resist change. Since EMS was sacrificed to the fire department to justify their existence, we "street people" have had the pleasure to see and experience FDNY up close and personal. So let's look at FDNY as you have never seen them before, but what we experience day in, day out.

Tom Reynolds and I responded to an "unconscious" in the projects on Sixty-second Street and Amsterdam Avenue in Manhattan, north of Roosevelt Hospital. We pulled up the same time as the housing police sector and went upstairs. The engine company was already there. The job was reportedly on the landing, off the hallway. As we entered, we saw the firemen kneeling in a circle around an eighteen-year-old blonde on the floor, forming a "Ring of Concern."

Their first aid was to provide the "Stare of Care." No they weren't doing anything but staring!

"Do you have Narcan?" one fireman asked as I stepped over the female with the drug bag. I smiled figuring it was nice to see them attempting to expand their limited vocabulary remembering they suffer from Toxic Brain Syndrome (Too much ego and not enough oxygen to the

119

remaining brain cells). "What's her respiration?" I foolishly asked.

"Two to four times a minute," a fireman proudly exclaimed.

"Don't you think you should be bagging her then?" I counted.

Normal breathing is twelve to eighteen times a minute. With respiration as low as hers, we needed to breathe for the patient with the BVM.

As CFRD (Certified First Responders), they should know this since I think pass the program at the CFRD program at the Academy they have to be able to count to at least twelve, without removing their boots.

"Don't worry," Tommy said, seeing the confusion on their faces, meaning, bag her and he'd explain the higher math concept of breathing later.

I approached the area by the window, to place the drug bag. The fire lieutenant shouted, "What the fuck is wrong with you two idiots? One says 'bag,' the other says, 'don't worry.'"

Without missing a beat, I hit him in the leg with the drug bag, thus backing him up giving me room to open it on the floor. Simultaneously I yelled, "Pick up!"— fire talk meaning clear the area. They realized it was EMS talk for "Get the fuck out of the area... now!"

Drawing up the Narcan, I heard a little hurt voice behind me.

"Don't you need us?"

"No, we are the paramedics. Besides, we have the cops here."

When I turned, Tom was smiling the cops were laughing, and the 'heroes' were gone. Pushing the Narcan-filled needle into her arm it shot through her body blocking the opium receptor sites from the heroin in the brain. Before Tom could open the BVM, the girl was awake, asking why we blew her high.

Narcan, also called Naloxone, is known on the streets as "Vitamin N."

The junkies hate it. Given too much, too fast, it gets them sick, as any new paramedic knows. It seemed I ruined Engine Forty-four's day also, which made my day. I wondered when they would learn that famous Paramedic idiom, 'breathing is fundamental.'

After the merger, AKA "the sacrifice," the fire gods—Thomas Von Essen, Fire Commissioner, Peter J. Ganci, Chief of the Department, and William M. Feehan, First Deputy Commissioner thought they knew how to run EMS, in general, and the paramedics in particular.

They decided paramedics should be in PRU (Paramedic Response Units), just like in the old days. It was the nineties and the Fire God knew he could run PRUs as well as the rest of EMS. But the twist was that each paramedic would ride with a lieutenant paramedic, just like on a fire truck.

The only unit that would have two paramedics was the HAZMAT Unit. At one time, this was a highly trained unit. Then the fire gods decided they did not like the idea of our people being better trained than their own. Thus, the "Mop and Glow Team," as we called them, became the guys who took the firemen's blood pressures, before and after they put on their self-contained suits.

Once again we changed our schedules to accommodate the new program.

On the plus side I had a great partner in Lieutenant Jo Ann Kovac. Paramedics were once again looking forward to coming to work to do ALS jobs and the PRU beat the hell out of the ambulance! But as with all things in EMS, now FDNY EMS the program was setup to fail.

First were the EMS officers who became officers to avoid patient care. They wanted more money yet nothing was said about the paramedic partner who carried their sorry assess through the call.

Secondly, Mr. Murphy from Murphy & Murphy appeared (What can go wrong will). The FDNY Gods let the same inept EMS Chiefs setup the program the way they crashed the first PRU Program. These buffoons did not add on an extra BLS unit to replace the ALS unit that became the PRU which had no transport capability! Thus the typical SNAFU (Situation Normal All Fucked Up) EMS environment nosed dived to FUBAR (Fucked Up Beyond Repair) before the first PRU hit the streets. What does this say for the Fire God's mentality? This is very similar to President Bush and the post 9-11 FBI (Famous But Inept). Nothing changed except the window curtains hiding the same inept idiots running the show within. Yeah these idiots were on top of their game the way General Custer was.

The program came to a crashing halt because of these shit-for-brain paper-pushers. As moral sank the public suffered even more than we. But in all fairness to EMS Chiefs FDNY could still outdo them for stupidity.

Some of us went to Fort Totten to get our worn-out short-sleeve shirts replaced. We were told that EMS people would no longer be issued short-sleeve, blue uniform shirts. Instead, we were issued polo shirts.

The only problem was that we would have to wait, because the genius, **a fireman** who ordered the shirts for the medics, **misspelled paramedic**. Hey, bravest yes, smartest, never and it gets worse!

At the website fdnysucksaol.com, it was reported that the Fire Department Institute (FDI) and Turner Publishing Company put out the NYC FD Millennium Edition. According to the FDNY, America entered World War II in 1942, not December 8, 1941, a day after the Japanese attacked Pearl Harbor.

Mistake, typo, you say? Well, according to the book, "EMS Dispatching is done from 1 Metro Tech." The idiots don't even know where their own EMS dispatchers are. Thus you could justify with ease how the hapless spineless EMS chiefs were outwitting the smoke-damaged mindless. In the game of brains and administrative efficiency, both were unarmed. All the while, Mayor Giuliani and the fire commissioner played with statistics. Robert Lederman, at **artistpresaol.com**, wrote a wonderful book on the great Mayor Giuliani. One of the interesting things he described was the **tampering with statistics**. Of course, it was denied.

The night was typically warm in Spanish Harlem, where we had been deployed. I pulled the bus over, when I spotted two cops standing on the corner, looking uneasy.

"Hey guys. What's up?" I asked.

"Not much," replied the petite and pretty Spanish police officer. Even in uniform, her physical beauty was apparent. But I saw the sadness in her large, dark eyes.

"So what's a nice girl like you doing in a place like this?" I asked.

"Hanging out," her voice couldn't hide anger. "There are no drugs in Spanish Harlem tonight," her voice crackled with authority, looking across the street at a drug deal going down. Even from here we could smell the reefer people were smoking.

"What?"

"Yeah, that's what I said. However, the lieutenant said there would be no drug collars tonight. Our statistics are too high."

"Makes you proud to be a cop, huh?"

"I came on this job three years ago hoping to make a difference. Now I just want out."

We spoke a little longer, with me wishing them both a safe tour before driving on. Thus the game of statistics was even played not only by the Fire Department, but by the Police Department as well, to project the mayor's agenda.

Mr. Lederman wrote, "To paraphrase a famous Zen saying, if a crime happens in New York City, but the police don't record it, did it really happen?" In this context, he was talking about the numerous sexual assaults that took place in Central Park, where the police reportedly did nothing. Well, not quite. They handed out an estimated seven hundred summonses for nonsexual attacks. If you think Mr. Lederman is incorrect about the good mayor, think again, and investigate. Talk about crime and organization wait till you read this next story.

Right after we were sacrificed to the Fire God, we had an "unconscious" in an SRO (Single Room Occupancy) hotel. It was a warm spring day, so standing outside the door, I could smell the ambiance of how really ripe our patient was. I banged on the door, no one responded. The superintendent didn't have a key, so we called for a police ESU to open the door. We were curtly informed to request "fire suppression" and they would "take the door." Gee, I love that macho fire talk.

A while later, the Bravest showed up. Two firemen, one in pants, the other in shorts, approached us from the elevator. Neither said hello, just,

"This the door?"

"Yep," I responded.

They looked at the door, feeling it.

"Don't worry, there's no fire there," one of the EMTs said as we all giggled.

Looking at us with disdain, they mumbled to each other, getting out their tools, and in great, dramatic Hollywood tradition, "took the door."

One would figure this was enough, right? Wrong. Someone must have told them there was a cameraman on the other side of the door. Thus as soon as they popped the door, they dropped their tools and both stormed in. John Wayne would have been proud. What they were going to do was beyond me but what happened next would have made the Russian Ballet Troupe proud. Without stopping, or letting their feet touch the floor, both spun around and almost knocked us over as they flew out of the room!

Casually leaning against the door buck, we observed what caused the macho heroes to flee. There before us was the patient's bloated body on the bed. Maggots were crawling where his eyeballs had been and a large rat sat on his chest, gnawing away at the dead meat. The hallway was filled with laughter as we heard our fire heroes puking down the hall.

Saint Marks is located in the East Village in Manhattan. In the early years of EMS it was quite a street. We found heroin overdoses, prostitution, and every craze applied to the human body there.

One Vietnam veteran, named "Saigon," sat on the corner, sometimes with his wife, begging until his asthma got so bad he would request a treatment. The street was wild with stabbings, pedestrians struck by cars, you name it. The shops had everything and anything, legal or not.

The energy on the street was phenomenal.

Between Second and Third Avenue sat a rehab center halfway up Saint Marks' tree-lined street. One day, a Basic unit got a call for an injury. They requested a backup to assist with the lift. Since Tom Reynolds and I were in the area, we volunteered. When we arrived, I saw the problem. First, the patient was a "quarter-pounder with cheese"—

Very, very, morbidly fat.

The BLS crew had, as usual, done the correct thing, securing him to a long board with a collar. Because of this guy's size and a two-floor carry-down on slippery steps, I called for another EMS unit. The dispatcher opted to call our fire suppression heroes. I sent the female EMT downstairs to greet the crew. Tom stood back and smiled, since he knew where this was leading.

The female EMT came to the landing with several firemen and their captain. The fireman took off their gloves and decreed, "Okay. You," pointing to the short female EMT, "take the head and we'll carry your bags."

I responded, "Wrong. She will do her share by helping carry in the center and you will get at the head of the patient."

The loudmouth fireman threw his gloves on the floor and continued, "We're not carrying anything but your bags."

Seeing the determination of his crew, the captain looked at me and said "We are here to assist you in carrying the bags. Not to do your job. And that's all. I'm the captain."

"Okay, captain," I countered. "You are a fire captain and I'm the paramedic. We do not need you to carry the bags, since you and your crew are not qualified to carry our bags. You are definitely unqualified, nor ever could do our job. Thus, you will do as I tell you."

He stared at me, neck veins popping out as Tommy smirked. I didn't have time for the stare down; besides, he would lose, so I pushed for the kill.

"If you are refusing to do as I say, then I will relieve you of the scene.

Next I will request police emergency service and I will see you in BITs."

Without waiting, I looked at the loudmouth and said, "You get at the head now." He looked at the captain and, of course, now attempted to lift from where he was standing. I reiterated, "The head! The thing on top of the shoulders," this time pointing to the head of the patient. Mr. Macho did as told.

Downstairs, the patient was placed in the back of the EMTs' bus. Tom climbed in, keeping the doors open, realizing the Bravest still didn't get it. As I stood outside, the captain came up to me with the penguins (firefighters).

"I'm a fire department captain and demand respect." Several of his penguins now closed the 'Circle of Concern' around me.

I guess this was supposed to be intimidating, but since we "EMS" people work the streets and they only work the red things, you know putting the wet stuff on red stuff I chuckled.

"I'm the paramedic. You and your men are here to *support every EMT and medic.*" Someone made a typical macho statement.

"Bucket fairies," I muttered as I stepped into the little 'gang.'

"Okay, let's get it straight so even *you* understand it," I said, raising my voice looking at the loudmouth. "You are the firemen. You are the fire captain. I am the paramedic. Thus, *I am the brains. You are the brawn.*

Got it?" They looked like they wanted a fight but were totally out of their element. The gang mentality certainly wasn't working.

"Hey, want to go for it? I guarantee there are a lot of EMS as well as PD who wouldn't mind assisting in a 10-13 call to kick what's left of your asses."

The first wise thing they did all day was turn and get on their little red truck.

At the station, Captain Stone was in an uproar. He wanted statements, since the fire captain had put in a complaint and, of course, the EMS civilian gods were panicking.

Stone called Tommy and I into his office asking what happened. We presented him with statements.

"I'm scheduled to have a meeting sometime next week over this issue! I want you two there."

Silence, silence always sends Stone into a panic, well especially from us.

He looked up and asked, "What's going on?"

"Oh, we'll be there. You can bet your sweet ass on that. In fact, I'm in the mood for a good throw down with those assholes." I turned to Tommy and smiled.

"Me too," Tommy said.

"Oh, no! Neither one of you will be there," Stone said.

"Hey, common cap! In a room with only them. Shit sounds like ass-kicking time to me," I said, Tommy echoing, sending Stone into hyper panic.

All that week we asked about the meeting. Only after the meeting, we were told Stone had made nice with the idiots. Would you expect less?

I'm sure neither the patient's best interest, nor our crew's, were put forward.

God forbid these heroes have any blemishes against them. Someone should check to see how many additional lawsuits the city acquired after they started the First Responder Program (CFR). Have DOI (Department of Investigation) open their files. Oh, I forgot, the mayor runs that bastion of justice. Interestingly enough *I contacted DOI* for information for this book under the Freedom of Information Act and you know what I received? A total of four (4) letters:

Letter one: **April 8, 2004**
"We are conducting a search of materials responsive to your request and will contact you."

April 22, 2004
"Please be advised that we are engaged in the process of searching for the material you requested. However, more time is needed."

May 7, 2004
"Please be advised we are still engaged in the process of searching for material you requested. However, more time is need..."

May 24, 2004
"A diligent search of Department of Investigation files has failed to uncover any materials responsive to your request"

I had asked about lawsuits against the city in regards to the CFR Program as well as criminal complaints of theft against FDNY and also the percentage on alcohol/drug rehab.

Staff writer Donald Bertrand wrote an interesting article in the Daily News on October 28, 1999, concerning Engine Company 273 and Ladder Company 129 of Flushing, New York. Aside from its more than four-minute response time to medical jobs, but less than a minute turnout time for fires, the house had other problems.

One firefighter reported to work saying he wished he had a run, so he could "fall off" the truck. He'd be eligible for LODI. He wasn't the brightest light in the marquee, since he didn't know the ins and outs of his disability package.

A *brother* made a 911 call to get his friend a run, so he could fall and legitimize his foot injury. Unfortunately, this shit for brains genius did not realize the police dispatcher could trace the call back to the firehouse. Once again, it proved testosterone and smoke do not equal smart.

Action was taken against the fireman who made the call, but everyone was silent about the other fireman. Perhaps they should look up the word "intent," then "fraud," or perhaps an endemic systematic problem of lies and cover-ups within the fire suppression side. We in EMS would call it theft of services. But at least these guys show up in front of the job.

Let's look at another engine's response, or lack of, in a ghetto area of the South Bronx.

Date: Feb. 3, 2001 ID 1800
Call Type: Unconscious
Location: 1230 Webster 3rd Floor Hallway
Assigned: Engine 050
15:51:07 Entry (When job came in)
15:51:07 Fire sent (8746) Sent to Fire
15:51:09 Fire Ack (Acknowledges)
03Feb0111549340103427070220252
15:51:17 Fire Assign 03Feb01154941 E050
(Engine 050)
15:51:28 Assigned (0899) 26W2 (Paramedic Unit)
15:51:32 Enroute
15:52:05 PDEMS (T60) Aided male 40–50 yr. old
sts (State) FC (Female Caller) anialist
15:53:39 Supplement PD (D11A) 04259209 Assigned
15:54:14 FIRE-ON SCENE 03Feb01155238 E050
(Engine 050)

16:02:07 Fire Clear 03Feb01160030 E050
16:02:25 ON SCENE (2831) 26W2 (PARAMEDICS)

Let's recap this job to see how these heroes served the public. A woman called in about an unconscious male, forty to fifty years old, in a third-floor stairwell.
Fire gets the job first. Remember, the mayor has to prove that fire can get there before EMS.
Engine 050 beat us to the call by 00:48:11. If you look at the numbers, it looks like they were on scene for close to eight minutes and then left eight seconds before we got there.
The funny thing is, *they were NEVER there!* We saw the engine pull out of their house, but never on Webster.

The police, PSA 7, were on scene for a while with two other officers.
They stated fire was never there.

We walked the three flights and waited for the PD dispatcher to contact the female caller. She came down and showed us where she had seen the individual stating *fire was never there.* There was no patient. Fire got credit for the run. They got extra money, I think it's over $5,000 a year in their paychecks as CFRs and they continued the big lie that this fantasy program was working.
If you think I am picking on Engine 050 too much, please forgive me. To show you what a sport I am, I'll be glad to introduce you to another unit. There is more than enough to go around.

Let's see the exploits of Engine 082.
Date: February 4, 2001
Call Type: Unconscious
Address: 1488 Hoe Ave. (Church)
Assign: Engine 082

12:36:38 PD Comp (T61) Fm Fl Mn-AT
Church-CB-Aided 28Y/O OPR 2291 (8643)
12:36:58 Entry (*643) FCS F28 UNC
12:36:58 Final Ack Cent to PD (8643)
12:36:58 Fire Sent (8643) Call sent to Fire
12:37:03 Fire Ack 04Feb 0112352301035273

12:37:15 FIRE ASSIGNED 04Feb01123537 E082
(Engine 082)
12:37:26 Assign (0899) 26W2 (Paramedics)
12:37:29 Enroute (2831) 26W2
12:40:43 Supplement-PD (D11A) 042E Assigned
12:41:00 FIRE ON SCENE 04Feb01123922 E082
(Engine 082)
12:42:15 On scene (2831) 26W2
12:42:48 Fire Clear 04 Feb01124109 E082
12:42:49 Fire Close 04 Feb 01124110

According to this, we have a female unconscious in a church. It would appear that Engine 082 was on the scene awaiting our arrival for over a minute. Remember, heart and brain cells die in four to six minutes.

Unloaded our equipment, one of the folks from the church asked if we needed help or wanted cars moved. He also looked up the block and asked, "Is that fire truck coming here also?"

"No sir," my partner answered. We proceeded to the patient.

Engine 82 was *never at the predominately black church in the South Bronx.*

The truth is evident to those of us who serve ghetto communities these firemen do not want to do the job for which they've been paid and tasked. They can hop on their trucks, get credit for the calls, and get the extra money—and not give a shit about the people. The people deserve better.

This would not have happened in Midtown Manhattan, where there are lawyers, cameras, and wealthy, influential residents.

Damn, again, the key question for me here concerns first and foremost the people we both serve. This book is not about bashing firefighters. This is about *their impact* on EMS units and ultimately on the lack of care patients receive from them. It took them longer than four minutes to respond to a medical job. The brain in the human body is in trouble after four minutes without oxygen. After six minutes, cells start to die. Thus these firemen were having a direct effect on the chances of patient survivability.

With response times like this, and after speaking to several of them since I visit Flushing everyday, I can attest they were neither of the caliber in education or devotion of Engine Company One in Manhattan. But again is there an endemic problem, or was this too an isolated incident of not caring about the public and "medical problems" if there were no red stuff to place the wet stuff on? Or does it go higher within the administrative culture that encourages this? Read the following and decide if there is a flaw in the macho culture of the "brotherhood."

During training periods out at the EMS Academy it's a time where paramedics and EMTs have an opportunity to not only update their knowledge and skills. It is also a time among peers to not only disseminate what they have learned through various cases of treating patients but also discuss "jobs" that bother them. I had the opportunity to hear firsthand of the following tragedy.

On January 19, 2001, a judge accused New York City attorneys and the fire department of attempting to cover up responsibility in a collision that killed a West Brighten woman and teenager. Now you can understand how come DOI claimed not to be able to find any information I requested. They were killed on July 13, 1996, by a fire truck responding to a downed electrical wire. The truck went through a red light at breakneck sped. The impact killed Kathy McAndrews, forty-eight, of West Brighten and sixteen-year-old Bridgette Flaherty of Concord. The truck driver of Ladder Eighty-three, housed at Jewett Avenue in Westerleigh, showed complete disregard or common sense as he recklessly careened through the wet and windy streets ramming into the driver's door of Mrs. McAndrews' at the corner of South Gannon and Bradley Avenues.

Conditions were dangerous because of the weather, yet the driver's arrogant ego did not give these civilians a chance. Mrs. McAndrews' sixteen-year-old daughter survived, no thanks to these heroes. Here's exactly what the Bravest did.

The fire department called for an "extensive investigation" and later the Bravest's spin meister stated, "The investigation has been concluded and no one acted in an inappropriate manner."

EMS crews were on the scene, protesting. The news report stated, "The medics complained about the quality of care administered by the firefighters to the woman and berated the firefighters' conduct." Also, they also singled out the fire captain of the unit, Rescue Five.

According to the medics on the scene, the firefighters removed the victims without providing the most basic precautions for preventing crippling or lethal injuries. Then they prevented the medics from trying to save the victims' lives.

This is nothing new with these bastards, as I was informed by Paramedic Lenny Hinden years earlier. In Queens, a fire truck was going for a Chinese dinner with lights and sirens and killed people in a car. They kept Lenny and his partner from getting to the patients. As you will recall in the Queens case, the gutless EMS chiefs tried to blame the medics. The scoundrels figured, no witnesses, no smudge on their image. But let's see how *this case developed.*

133

As the medics tried to get to the patients, another unit responded and a shoving match started. At this point, a female EMT was physically picked up and moved out of the way by one of the Bravest.

Once again, our medical section did a review and stated, "The firefighters adequately administered first aid and no disciplinary action would be taken against the captain."

Finally, the fire department safety battalion investigated the collision and found "no fault with the crew of Ladder Eighty-three." Then the bastards blamed the deceased, Mrs. McAndrews, for the crash, clearing their own men.

Thanks to love and determination, Mr. William McAndrews had his day in court. His attorney, Michael J. Kuharski of Kuharski and Levitz, did his homework and presented the case to the people. With the information in the open, the people were not fooled. Nor could the spin meisters hide what came out at the trial.

Fact, Firefighter Greg Callaghan, who was behind the wheel of the fire truck, gave conflicting accounts of what happened.
Fact, after the collision, instead of stopping like any reasonable person would do, he backed up. This did more damage to the car.
Fact, the safety battalion stated that Ladder Eighty-three had stopped at the red light.
Fact, an off-duty fireman witnessed the collision and stated that Ladder Eighty-three never stopped or even slowed down.
Fact, the witness's statement was never included in the official fire department report.
Fact, those EMS people were called to court.
Facts, the people of the jury saw right through the Bravest and saw the incident for what it was. It was such a despicable show. New York Supreme Court Justice Alan Lebowitz went after the fire department as well as the City Corporation Counsel (the department that handles cases against the city)

for its "callous attitude" in attempting to cover up the incident.

"I'm appalled by the testimony," he said and later went on to state that he had **"never heard such fabrication as I did from the firefighters."**

The McAndrews family was awarded $10,801,945. The Bridgette Flaherty case was settled with the city also.

It would appear that the New York City Fire Department has the same belief perfected by Stalin, if you keep telling the same lie over and over again and sprinkle it with photos of heroes, soon everyone will believe it.

I just wish to put the Fire God of Puzzle Palace (9Metro Tech) on notice. The public may be fooled, but the EMS people aren't. I guess that was why former Commissioner of Public Affairs Mr. Regan told EMS Lieutenant Vinny Hanlon that he did not want people from outside agencies riding as observers on EMS units. His exact words were "with those disgruntled EMS people."

***

It was a cold, rainy, blustery winter day as we pulled out of Battalion 26 in the South Bronx. It amazed me that such a cold, depressing structure was considered appropriate for EMS crews by health professionals. The "Little Tin House" was essentially that—a tin garage, wedged between two buildings, that was currently acting like a "big ice box." With the ability to fit only three ambulances, one behind the other, bumper on bumper, the whole place would rapidly fill with a blue mist as the diesel engines were started. Diesel fuel has been scientifically proven to contain over forty deadly carcinogenic elements positively linked to everything from asthma, high blood pressure, cardiac problems, to cancer!

If you were the third unit, and we were, you'd cough and gag your brains out. The only consoling thought for me was that the officer's desk, the guys entrusted to take care of us, was right next to the front door and directly adjacent to the first vehicle receiving the brunt of the poisonous deadly fumes from all three units. Still nothing was done to improve the air quality, or even paint the facility to psychologically help crews' distress during change of shift before heading home. The structure itself mimicked most facilities in its drab, lifeless, depressing colors. Rats, the four-, not two-legged ones, were common in the tight, lifeless, stoically lit locker room. Concerning time, the only time the officers wanted to see a unit back at the facility was during tour change. How different it was with the firemen, I thought.

The New York Times ran an article, "Firemen, Call Your Decorators" by John Leland, who wrote, "For the 21 firefighters in Engine Company 210, the firehouse is much more than a place of business. 'This is like my second home,' said Robert Labas, one of the firefighters mopping the first floor bathroom. Firefighters spend long shifts in domestic idle, punctuated by momentary encounters with chaos. They cook their own meals on the big Vulcan stove in restaurant quality kitchens. They sleep in the dormitory upstairs. They work out on the treadmills [not one, mind you, but several], in the workout area."

In another article in The Daily News, Deputy Mayor Marc Shaw called FDNY a "bastion of inefficiency" where firefighters are "hanging around, doing nothing 95% of the time."

In all fairness, firefighters, when fighting fires or conducting rescue missions, have an extremely physically demanding job, and there is not one EMS EMT or paramedic who would deny this. Having said that, one must also acknowledge the statistical evidence discovered by Local 2507. The study showed dramatically that firefighters are out of their house only four hours in a twenty-four-hour day. To reiterate, in all fairness it must also be understood that both jobs are diametrically different. Firefighters operate from a static box location; in other words, they respond to 99.9 percent of fires within their assigned area. EMS operates on a flow system, which is more dynamic.

An example is that although I and my partner Jack Ng are pulling out of Bellevue on 26th Street and First Avenue in Manhattan, if the call volume dictates, then we are redeployed to 218th Street and Tenth Avenue, in the Bronx.

This, because of poor administrative planning for staffing units, happens often. On more than one occasion we were the "only medic unit," according to the dispatcher, pulling out of Bellevue at 6 p.m. on a hot summer's night and given a "cardiac arrest" at 218th Street. The sheer volume of vehicular traffic made it a death sentence for the patient, even had a proficient CFR unit gotten to the scene in under four minutes.

There are times when an engine company is redeployed, but when this happens they occupy the quarters of the engine they are replacing.

Whereas EMS crews sit on a street corner, until a call comes in, for either eight or sixteen hours. Sitting in a vehicle with diesel fumes enveloping the public and crew is bad enough, health wise. Blood clots form from extended periods of sitting, as any medical professional or airline stewardess will tell you.

Also, no one wants to be sitting for sixteen hours next to the active computer we have mounted between the crew members. Having said that, I know street deployment is the best way to serve the public for EMS.

A setup like those of the firemen would not work. But there is no excuse for not providing decent facilities when they come in for the change and restock, or clean sleeping quarters and showers for those working endless mandated tours.

It is a joke to talk about the facilities the Fire God has promised and delivered. The Harlem facility, which was praised by the mayor and his Fire God, had more leaks than the Titanic. And you can tell me Mr. Giuliani and his Fire God aren't masters of deception? Where were the 'investigative reporters' instead of the cellophane entertainers like Dan Rather? Why doesn't someone look into the contractor who was paid handsomely by the Giuliani administration to build the facility? Follow the money and it will prove to be better reading.

Daily News Bronx Bureau Chief Bob Kappstatter reported, "Public Advocate Mark Green's office uncovered a consultant's report for the fire department. It disclosed above average levels of lead, mercury, arsenic, and other toxic substances in the subsoil at the proposed EMS site (West 230th Street and Tibbett Avenue in the Bronx). The site bordered Public School 37 and Kennedy High School." The article continued,

"Green said besides lead, mercury, and arsenic, the study of the subsoil at the site found elevated levels of benzo (a)pyrene and chrysene, both possible carcinogens."

What was the response of the Fire God, Fire Commissioner Von Essen? "We believe that the environmental concerns raised by the parents are not problematic." The report stated that children had to be evacuated from their school after "lead dust was discovered in two air ducts. The dust was believed to have been churned up by construction work at the garage site (EMS facility)."

A fire department source stated that the fire commissioner was "frustrated with the delays and near certainty of longtime litigation that was going to take place."

For his part, Green "congratulated" the fire commissioner for his decision "to put the health and safety of children at PS 37 first." I never did like that two-faced, gutless advocate, Green.

Perhaps because I am known as a very sensitive guy, I am missing something here. The Fire God didn't see a problem, but the parents, damn those minorities and consulting firm did. I bet this firm won't do more work for the fire department. The people in the South Bronx are abused enough with diesel fumes, which I firmly believe have created the worst asthma site in the United States.

Neither the Fire God nor Mr. Green said a damn thing about not moving EMS into the facility.

A firehouse at One Hundred Eighty-third Street and Jerome Avenue in the Bronx was listed as "uninhabitable" for the firemen and closed. So a new facility was built.

Then the Fire God tried to move EMS units into the old hellhole. Once again, the chiefs demonstrated no spine as they followed orders. Thanks to President Pat Bahnken, of our local, a quick stop was put to it. However, another "new" EMS facility was opened and crews moved in even as crews continue to complain about dangerous poor air quality.

FDEMS Battalion 18 sits next to a plastics factory! Crews still get sick, yet nothing gets done. FDNY firefighters were moved out of yet another facility because it had "uninhabitable conditions." EMS was moved into the rehabbed structure, now home of FDEMS Battalion 19. Water still leaks, mold still grows. In fact, to date an unknown fungus has never been cleaned and crews are sick.

These are just several examples of how the Fire God, and his spineless cronies, the civilian EMS chiefs, and the EMS Medical Director have put crews in harm's way by moving EMS people into toxic and uninhabitable facilities.

The rain increased as Angelo and I received a call for an "asthmatic on the corner." Angelo muttered as we attempted to see out the window that was freezing up. The crew compartment was cold because the heater was blowing a teasing "warm" breeze. Historically, EMS had ordered the crews to "remain in service" with or without heat or air conditioning as long as the "patient compartment" had these functions. The degree of these "functions" did not matter because we were given heavy gray "horse blankets" to keep the patient warm. But that was then, the old EMS of the Bobby Becker days. This was now and we were part of the greatest fire department in the world. The windshield wipers scraped harmlessly across the thickening forming ice. With my toes numbed, I opened the window, trying to help Angelo navigate to find our patient. The wet, freezing rain-snow-sleet combination started to soak both my uncovered exposed head and non-waterproof turnout coat. I would like to know why we were issued "turnout coats" that are not raincoats? We were told to bring them in to get them sprayed with Scotchgard. Needless to say, this band-aid solution wasn't working. Why is it, if we wanted hoods, we would have to buy them, as well as pants?

The whole purpose of the turnout coat was protection against BBP (blood-borne pathogens). What happens when we kneel next to the patient?

Why was a newly designed raincoat given to the former female ALS coordinator in Manhattan, a.k.a. EMS Command Chief Robert Mc-Cracken's aide and Captain Mark Stones 'friend'? Why not test it with the workers, not the pencil pushers, kneepad expert clerks, and jerks? Why have we not received the appropriate gear in the first place? Perhaps Mr. James Geraci, MSU director, could answer this.

I cursed as we exited the vehicle, stepping into a cold, wet slush that soaked right through my FDNY-issued boots. We were issued boots with poor support. I was hurt and went to BHS. Nothing was done, so I went back to Bellevue Hospital and saw Dr. Thomas R. Penny of Podiatric Medicine and Surgery. I had, among other things, falling arches from the heavy loads we carry and the non-arch-supporting boots. It took two painful shots of cortisone and custom-formed inserts to relieve the problem.

When other EMTs and paramedics complained to the fire department about the boots, they were told, "It's because you are overweight." I am certainly not overweight.

Angelo and I approached a mother holding her slumping son. Immediately, we got the boy and mother into the back of the bus out of the rain. As the twelve-year-old fought to breathe, we administered medicine via a nebulizer. The mother informed us he had a history of asthma and a "heart problem." Angelo, after evaluation, encouraged the boy to take deep breaths and hold it so the medication would work. As we continued to evaluate the patient, I attempted to do an EKG of his heart to better understand the "heart problem." After opening two brand-new packages of EKG pasties, we finally had some that adhered to the patient as we attempted to keep him warm.

Satisfied with the printout, we attempted to keep him warm by wrapping him in the newly issued FDNY blankets. Our breath frosted as we spoke in the lukewarm air that we were waiting to heat up. That would take another hour at least. The boy shivered, so I took off my partially drenched, useless turnout coat and placed it around him over the two useless, paper-thin blankets.

With him now sitting more erect and able to speak, we headed toward Lincoln Hospital.

If you want to sell something to the City of New York, you need to be the lowest bidder. I would like to see the IRS audit of Mr. James Geraci, now MSU director. Mr. Geraci was anything but a loved dispatcher. It was rumored that, one night, while he sat at the communications board, cigarette in hand he set his wig on fire. Then he became MSU (Medical Supply Unit) director and we have been complaining ever since.

We also heard he had received 'incentives' for saving the fire department money. If so, I'd like to know how much? Medics have complained about the cheap EKG pasties as well as the cheap catheters we use for the longest time.

We hit a new low with EMS Command order 2000-57, issued September 20, 2000, concerning blankets. We had used heavy, gray "horse blankets." They were big and thick, keeping the patient warm. Then we were issued wafer-thin, white blankets with FDNY printed on them in bold blue letters. These blankets are a disgrace and disservice to the public.

I'd like to know how much Mr. Geraci has made while saving the Fire God's money? Or is it just a rumor? If only a rumor, why is he allowing such crap into the field?

As for audits, I call upon the IRS, or any other federal agency concerned with waste and fraud, to answer why the 1996 report by State Comptroller H. Carl McCall has had **no**

141

impact on the way the New York City Fire Department wastes money? The report gave a new meaning to incompetence concerning billing.

An article dated November 1, 2000 in the New York Post reported a $39 million loss by NYFD in the billing area. Since Deputy Commissioner Frank Gribbon, who spoke for the fire department, did not dispute the findings, why was this incompetence allowed to continue?

What was the governor of New York doing? We know what Giuliani was doing. As stated earlier, he cut HHC's (Health and Hospital Corpo-ration's) budget by millions one year and gave us to the fire department the next.

Of every $100 dollars the city spends, $3.46 is spent on the fire department and $0.32 on EMS. Even a report from the Citizens' Budget Commission used the words "resource underutilization" and "inefficiency" to describe the fiasco of the New York City Fire Department. But, really, how efficient is inefficiency in FDNY? We already know fires in New York are down dramatically. But to answer inefficiency, we need to answer the following question. How many firemen does it take to change two tires on an ambulance sitting in the middle of the Korean Day Parade?

Paramedic Arty Gonzales and I were parked at Thirty-fourth Street and Broadway in Manhattan right across the street from Macy's. It was another glorious, mellow day in Manhattan as we leisurely left the vehicle and went to get some well-deserved breakfast. An ever so faint smell of flowers from the local garden embraced by a warm breeze tantalized our noses. Caretakers of the small bastion of greenery and vibrant colors within the concrete jungle wished us a good morning before returning to watering the kaleidoscope of colorful plants. Tourists were just starting to leave their hotels and a few New Yorkers were out for the newspapers and Starbucks Coffee. The sun glistened off Macy's as we made our way to Paxs. As usual, I joked with my friend to put his shirt tale into his pants. Yes indeed, the day was new and peaceful. I wondered what it held in store for us.

When we returned, I noticed that the unit was sitting on an angle. By now, you realize the job is not on the level, but the bus should be. Sure enough, we had not one, but two flats on the passenger side. Arty got on the radio after securing his breakfast on the council and informed the dispatcher that we had two flats and needed the fire department tire truck to respond.

That should do it, right? Wrong. We are not allowed to request the tire truck or roadside repair. We can carry narcotics, use all sorts of lethal medications on you or your family members. We can put a tube down your throat, or stick a needle into your chest to help you breathe. But only a supervisor can request roadside assistance. Talk about a lack of efficiency here. But, whatever happened, I had full faith that FD could and would supersede our pundits in inefficiency.

But that was just fine by Arty and me, as we started to enjoy our breakfast while waiting for an EMS supervisor to tell the dispatcher we had two flats. We waited and waited. Finally, a tired Lieutenant Espeut showed up. Without getting out of his vehicle, he confirmed the job requesting the tire truck, before going in for the tour change.

About two blocks down from us, the Koreans were gathering for their parade. Unfortunately, the route would be through our section of Broadway. As a burly, good-natured police sergeant approached, other cops were putting up the blue barricades for the parade.

"Hey guys. Want to move this, please?" he asked.

"We'd like to, but we have two flats. The tire truck is on the way."

"Okay," said the sergeant, walking away.

Quite a while later, the fire department tire truck showed up. After finishing his paperwork, the mechanic got out of his vehicle and approached.

"Hi guys. Which tire?"

"Hi, two on that side," Arty responded.

In astonishment, "Two tires?"

"Yeah, that's what I told Central," Arty said.

"I'm not sure I have two tires."

"Whatever," I said looking at my watch. "Let's wait another ten minutes. Then we'll get some lunch."

Yes, gentle reader, it was almost lunch time and our tour started at seven in the morning. It took the guy another several more minutes to realize he had the tires and finally remove them from the storage compartment of his truck.

After getting our lunch, we returned to the bus. The tire mechanic was standing next to the driver's door, looking confused.

"What's up?" Arty asked, getting into the driver's seat with his food.

"There's a slight problem," he uttered, still confused, now looking at the sea of colorful uniforms and flags as the Koreans started to gather for their parade.

"Wrong size tire?" I queried.

"Oh, no!" he uttered in utter shock. "My compressor isn't working. I was in a rush and they told me everything worked on the truck."

No compressor, no power tools. No power tools no can change the tires.

"Well, we sure hope you come up with a solution," Arty said, diving into his food.

"Yeah, we get off at three and aren't looking for overtime," I added.

The guy went to make a phone call. When he came back he told us "they" were sending a mechanic from Brooklyn to fix the compressor.

Hey, it was now lunchtime do you really think we cared?

Well, the sergeant was getting a little edgy as he walked over.

"How's it going?"

"Pretty good food here," I said.

"No, I mean the flats. The captain wants to know what's happening."

"Sir, you can ask the gentleman standing back there," I said, pointing with my fork to the rear of the truck as I continued to eat. A short time later, the mechanic came up, complaining about the sergeant, saying he threatened to tow us away.

"Hey, that's cool," I said. The mechanic ran for the phone as Arty let the dispatcher know we were still here.

Returning from his phone call, the mechanic proudly proclaimed,

"Help is on the way! Don't worry," while cautiously spying the police sergeant across the street. Seems the "mechanic" was a fireman on "light duty" for over five years and evidently came up with a solution to the problem.

"Whatever," we said laughing as if either Arty or I cared.

We watched Engine One, lights on, siren blaring, head up Sixth Avenue, wondering where the "cardiac" call was. A short time later, they pulled alongside us. By and far, these guys were the best in the city to work with on medical jobs, but fix a compressor? So this was his idea, to call his brothers? So here we sat, one FDNY ambulance, Engine Company, firemen walking around in bunker pants, an FDNY tire truck, even more Koreans, tourists, spectators, and an annoyed, escalating to frustrated, NYPD Sergeant.

After what seemed a half-hour, Arty and I returned with another cup of coffee and were conversing with two lovely young girls from England when the closed-door meeting of the "minds" broke as we heard them request yet another engine over the radio. Hey, you know what happens when smoke fills those synaptic spaces between brain cells. Once the smoke hits the brain you are never the same, and these boys were certainly proving to be hypoxic, *slow on the uptake here.*

But, understanding their medical problems and being full of compassion, Arty looked over at me. "Let's try some place different for dinner," he said, chuckling.

In the end, it took a fire department tire truck, two engine companies (five men per truck with two officers), an

EMS supervisor who had to confirm it, and a police sergeant to threaten to have the vehicle towed away, to finally change two tires. It was a short day for us. Arty went to work at his second job, well rested, and the Koreans had a great parade.

The fire gods instituted a "promotional exam" required to become a firefighter. Not even the EMTs felt it was a promotion, rather a demotion, to become a firefighter. Still, considering the money firemen receive and the perks, some of the guys wanted to switch. I looked at it as a plus for us in that it would mean more of our people infiltrating over there. With such stealth moves perhaps one day the average firefighter would know the difference between a Ford 4x4 and a 4x4 bandage.

After the gods claimed it was a promotional exam, they decided to discriminate against age. The union felt it was indeed discrimination and drew up the appropriate paperwork. They went to Captain Green who ran NYFD EEO unit. As the union tried to serve the office the EEO complaint, all of the firemen, every last one of them, stood there with their hands in their pockets, refusing to accept the EEO, more content to play with their hose than do what was right.

This was all smoke and mirrors by the Fire God to improve their disgraceful statistics concerning minorities.

On December 20, 2000, as Angelo and I pulled out of Battalion 26 in the South Bronx, I knew our tour would be interesting, to put it mildly. I decided to keep tabs on the calls, the ones fire was assigned, but even I wasn't ready for this shock.

We were assigned a "cardiac arrest" at 3468 Park Avenue with a cross of One Hundred Sixty-eighth Street. The information on the computer read as follows:

13:54:13 Entry (Dispatcher 8652) CSP (Call says patient) M(male) Elderly. Dialysis patient NOT BREATHING in main waiting area.

13:54:17 Sent to PD (Police Department)
13:54:17 Sent to Fire (8652) Call sent to FIRE
13:54:20 Fire AKA [Acknowledges]
13:54:21 Fire Assign (Assigned)
13:54:29 PDEMS (T65) FC (Female caller) Sts(states) aided was choking. They ARE
DOING CPR
13:54:43 Assigned (0899) 26W2 [This is my unit and my partner is Paramedic Angelo
Morales (2831).]
13:55:23 Assist (0899) 26F2
[This is a Basic unit with EMTs Correa (2743) and Caballero (2249), both very competent EMTs.]
13:55:45 Supplement PD (Police Department) assigned 042H assigned
13:56:21 26W2 Enroute (2831)
13:56:38 26F2 Enroute (2849)
13:56:38 FIRE ONSCENCE 20, Dec. 00135718 ENG (ENGINE) 050
13:57:29 26F ONSCENE
14:00:02 Fire CLEAR E (Engine) 050
14:00:02 Fire CLOSE
14:02:06 26W2 ONSCENE

We can see how well the mayor utilized the fire department to serve the citizens and taxpayer. The call came into the system and was assigned the fire department Engine 050 first. This was based on the premise to reiterate that they operate out of a fixed firehouse and, as such, should get there first. It took them two minutes and seventeen seconds to get on the scene. Pretty good, but then it fell apart.

They were on the scene before the first EMS unit, but they *never got off the truck*. Brain cells die in four to six minutes and these guys waited for close to a minute before the first EMS unit arrived.

From the time they pulled up until they cleared the scene was four minutes. Brain cells are dying and what the fuck were these idiots doing? Collecting extra money as certified first responders!

Thanks to the good work of EMTs Correa and Caballero, the sixty-three-year-old gentleman survived. He had finished dialysis at a clinic and was eating, when he choked on a roast beef sandwich. A nurse did the Heimlich maneuver, abdominal thrust, and he expelled the meat.

This nurse had it together, as she stood next to the patient with a BVM in case she had to breathe for him. Interestingly, but not surprising, **_not one doctor_** came to help the patient.

The next day, December 21, 2000, proved even more interesting in the land of Fire Follies. On this day, Angelo and I were assigned 890 Faile Street with a cross of Senica. The job was a "difficult breather" Segment 2 on a three-year-old asthmatic child.

10:16 26W2 Assigned
10:18:10 Assist 03B2 This is a Basic unit with EMTs Dohert (3207) and Rodriguez-Arenal
(2724) Both from Battalion 55
10:20:02 03B2 ONSCENE
10:23:12 26W2 ONSCENE

The three-year-old did not need ALS intervention and was only dealing with a cold. The professional EMTs of 03B2 cleared us off the scene. What has this got to do with the fire department?

It was a cool morning, and as I sat in the bus reviewing the job, "a three-year-old in imminent trouble" according to the text, guess what I saw _directly_ across the damn street? There sat a firehouse at Faile and Senica, right across the fucking street! **_The nearest firehouse was never assigned yet it was a priority call for a child no less!_**

In all my years on the streets, the only "save" was a twelve-year-old in arrest secondary asthma with Jack Ng. As any paramedic or emergency room doctor will tell you, once kids crash, most of the time, it's over. They get to go into the cold earth, not to summer camp. Yet certified first responders pick and choose their jobs. But more on that later, the morning is still young, let's see what else happened.

Later in the day, we were assigned a job at 965 Tinton Avenue with a cross of East One Hundred Sixty-fifth Street. All day, we did jobs that *__fire never responded to__*, so we weren't surprised when we read the text on the computer.

"Anaphylaxis, Engine on scene."

When someone has an anaphylactic reaction, it is a life-threatening emergency. The patient needs what paramedics carry. That includes large-bore IV needles to give fluid and epinephrine administered either by a shot in the arm, by IV, or down the endotracheal tube, if we have to intubate. The patient also needs a shot of Benadryl to stop the histamine release. There may be a need for cardiac monitoring and more medications. What the patient does not need is the 'Ring of Concern' providing the 'Stare of Care'.

In this case, it was a nine-year-old little girl. Angelo and I decided we would have the last laugh on the commissioner's troops. We quickly grabbed our gear, donned thick, blue gloves and infectious masks over our faces, and entered the building.

The stench of newly donated urine cut right through our masks. As we got off the elevator, we walked past the firemen standing in the dank hallway. One had an oxygen bag, another a lantern, yet another a tool for gaining entry or for protecting themselves. Well, at least they were standing in front of the correct apartment, I chuckled to myself.

The burnt smell from their bunker gear filled the hallway as one fireman smugly stepped forward, pronouncing; "The kid is allergic to the cat."

We went on the offense real fast.

"Excuse me," Angelo said, pushing past them, knocking on the apartment door.

"What's going on here?" the confused-looking, rum-faced, emaciated lieutenant asked.

At this point, there was alarm in his voice. Ignoring his question, I queried in a raised voice, "What the hell are you guys doing here?"

"Uh, it's an allergic reaction, we were told," one firefighter uttered.

"Well, first off, if it is anaphylaxis, exactly what can you do? Do you carry Epi? Diphenhydramine, Benadryl, or fluids?" I love confusing them with names.

"Uh, no, but . . . ," the officer remarked, totally baffled.

I cut him short. "Listen. We got the update as a very contagious disease, allergic reaction. I suggest you guys get out of here now!"

"That's right," Angelo uttered. "Think we enjoy getting dressed up like this?" he asked, stepping into the apartment.

With this, I stepped into the apartment, closing the door on several firemen who tried to spy the situation. The smirk was now off the face of the fireman who first remarked about the cat.

Inside, we busted a gut laughing, which I'm sure the "Bravest" heard.

The mother of the child informed us this was the first time she'd ever called 911.

"What are you here for?" she had asked as five firemen attempted to enter the apartment, only getting as far as the narrow vestibule area.

The lieutenant attempted to explain, but was curtly cut off as she demanded, "What the hell are you going to do, hose us down?" before throwing them out of the apartment.

Raging fires they deal well with, most of the time. However, even they realized the five of them were no match for a raging Puerto Rican mother in the South Bronx. As Mom told the story, we all laughed hysterically, tending to her daughter, Zeina, a true Princess Warrior who, by the way, was not having an anaphylactic reaction, nor was allergic to the cat.

Date: 1-31-2001 ID 2133
Call type: Difficulty Breathing

The call was for a sixty-five-year-old female who was assaulted. According to the computer text she was complaining of chest pain, with a history of lung cancer and triple bypass surgery. The text stated she was in the lobby of the building.

Address: 1252 West Farms Road, South Bronx
Assigned: Engine 82

Turning onto the block, we saw the engine, from several blocks away, stopped in front of the building. The ELI (Emergency Light Indicator) as we call the fire truck, just sat there. Not one of them got their asses off the truck to check the lobby for this elderly female. In fact as we pulled up behind them, they drove away without even an acknowledgement of our presence— complete apathy.

After parking, we grabbed the gear and walked between the cars to the old, steel-grated lobby door. I attempted to open it but it was locked, its grimy, worn knob having seen better days. Peering through the dirty, water-stained window, I saw the elderly woman holding her chest across the ancient thirty-foot lobby. Angelo banged on the door while I rang the door bells. Realizing someone was at the door, the old lady looked up and called, "Please! Someone help me!"

"We're here, hon." I called. "We'll get to you in a minute."

Angelo took out his knife to try to jimmy the door, nothing.

"Those fuckin' assholes!" I said, looking at him. "She's holding her chest, think we'll need to call them back."

"I can walk to the door," she called in a weaker, strained voice, attempting to rise off the ancient radiator.

"NO! Stay right there and we will get to you," I called back, not wanting her to exert herself, possibly passing out from a heart attack on the floor. Angelo continued to frantically work the lock when suddenly a young man appeared in the lobby.

"Yo! Please open the door for us," I called. The kid looked at us, then at the old lady, and walked away. "Mother fucker!" I yelled kicking the door.

Within a few seconds, as I reached for the radio, ready to demand ESU (Emergency Service Unit) of the Police Department, as opposed to the engine, an older male came to investigate the loud crash as I kicked the door and let us in.

"Thanks, man!"

"Anytime for EMS," he muttered, walking away, glancing at the old lady.

After a fast initial evaluation, we took her by stair chair to the bus. As we continued our evaluation, the story unfolded. She had been accused of stealing then savagely beaten in the chest and body by an Indian security guard in his early twenties who towered over her. After the assault, the woman called the cops, then her daughter. A foot cop from the Forty-first Precinct responded. He told her, "Unless you have broken bones I can see, I can't do any paperwork and arrest these guys. So why don't you just go home."

"I need EMS," she pleaded.

"Call when you get home," he coldly said, walking to talk to the owner whose son was the security guard.

With chest pain increasing, and realizing she was not going to receive help from the officer, the elderly five-foot-two-inch-tall grandmother mournfully walked unsteadily out of the store, holding the wall of the building. The four blocks were long as the terrifying chest pain increased.

Several times the old lady stopped to catch her breath, depositing crimson spots on the dirty concrete sidewalk from blood issuing from a lacerated lip. Her body was wracked with pain from the assault. Finally, after what seemed an hour, she made it to her building, several blocks away. Once inside, unable to go any further, she hysterically called her daughter through the now excruciating pain.

As we worked her in the back of the bus, she sobbed.

"Why didn't you call us from the store location?" Angelo asked.

"Because I was ashamed that you would think I stole something, I never did, ever."

A knock came on the door as her daughter, extremely distraught, arrived. The girl had gone to the store and the officer said he was doing the paperwork. He claimed not to know where her mother was. In the back of the bus, the daughter listened to the complete story, choking back the rage.

I heard a knock on the bus's door. Two police officers from the Forty Second Precinct asked what happened, thinking the assault took place at this location.

"Oh, that's in the Four-One," he remarked.

Suddenly a banshee's howl erupted from the daughter as a cataclysmic typhoon of rage furiously crashed down upon all in the bus.

"You're cops, right! But white cops and we're black, so it's the same old shit!"

"Miss, we're . . ."

Before he could finish, "Fuck you!" she screamed, followed by a horrific, thunderous, primordial wail. "Get out of here and leave us alone!"

Thunderbolts of lightning leapt from her eyes. We could see and feel the pain from her very soul. The girl's face was grotesquely contorted in untold rage from a lifetime of abuses.

"Give me a minute guys?" I asked, closing over the door as they waited outside, having not heard the complete story.

I had watched the exchange and realized both sides were listening, but not hearing. The two hardworking cops were trying to do a job.

The girl, seated, coiled, and realizing she wasn't ready yet, "I'll be right back," I said, stepping out, allowing the energy from her outburst to finish draining her of fight. Speaking to both officers, I filled them in completely. Both were outraged and felt the same as we did about the other officer, who never even called for a bus, even though the lady said she was injured. These cops were sincere in wanting to help the old woman and her daughter.

Once back inside the bus, "Okay, let's talk," I said softly but firmly. "Coming off with an attitude and going into defensive mode isn't helping one bit."

The mother interrupted, "I'll be fine. I just don't want any more trouble. I'm not going to the hospital."

"Young lady," Angelo said, holding up the EKG (which was fine, but it got both mother and daughters attention), "You are going to the hospital."

They both looked at me as I nodded.

Looking at the daughter, I said, "I want you to take a deep breath in. Good; hold it, now let it out slowly. Good, two more times."

She shot a glance at her mom who nodded her approval. After the third exhalation, I saw the stress leave her shoulders as they slumped forward. Her face muscles softened as the fiery storm left beautiful, clear, brown eyes.

"Now young lady, I'm calling the guys back in and you will explain in detail what happened to Mom." She nodded in total capitulation. "These guys both Angelo and I have seen before—they're good."

"And on your side," Angelo echoed.

"I'm sorry, I . . ."

"We know, and so do they. So listen, but above all else hear what they are saying, okay?" I said, running my hand over hers. I opened the door as she wiped a tear away.

"Okay, guys. Both young ladies would like to talk to you." Both women giggled.

As the first cop stuck his head in, "Is it safe now?"
The two women were laughing.

"I'm really sorry," the girl started, glancing over to me.

Both officers graciously explained what should be done and what they could, and could not, do.

After listening and with both parties moving beyond the stereotypes of uniform and race they heard each other. The officers explained to the daughter that if the other cop did not do his job, she could call them.

He gave her a card with a number on it. "We'll go to bat for your mom and you."

As I stepped out to thank the cops, Angelo wisely convinced the woman to go to Lincoln Hospital instead of Bronx Lebanon. I smiled, realizing it was an honor to work with Angelo Morales. Besides, there had been enough trauma; physically and psychologically, for one day. As we rode, I monitored the patient and spoke to the daughter.

"You saw two white cops and your defenses went up. You went off on them. They, on the other hand, were looking at a black female in the South Bronx, whose attitude won't give them a chance. Thus they went into a defensive mode." She intently nodded.

"Because of who these two cops are, they persisted in trying to help you. I spoke to them outside. They knew exactly what the first cop did. We all do. They knew it was wrong and wanted to see him nailed, since he makes their jobs harder." I paused, continuing, "We need to stop seeing our uniqueness, you black, them white, and look at our birthright of love, where we find a common bond."

"Thank you," she softly whispered, a sparkle back in two big, brown eyes, as a warm tender smile graced her face.

Concerning Engine Eighty-two, they got the credit for the run and the extra money in their paycheck as CFRs. But they shortchanged an old lady who needed them. Once again, I'll reiterate that the woman was black, not that it should matter, but it does. On more than one occasion, I have seen active racial discrimination take place by way of Engine Companies in the ghetto and on two occasions to two friends, outstanding EMS supervisors.

In one incident there was a reported fire at NYU Hospital on First Avenue and Thirty-third Street. I was standing with Lt. T. Hiller who, aside from being a gentleman and friend, was the Incident Commander.

A battalion chief walked up and started giving me the rundown and asking what resources I had available.

"Excuse me, sir, but this is Lt. Hiller. He's in charge."

"Yeah I know," he said curtly, "But I'm talking to you."

I felt like shit for "T": "No, you are not talking to me," I said. "If you are talking to anyone, it will be my officer."

With this, the chief strode away.

The next incident took place at 59th Street and Columbus Circle on a reported "gas attack, with numerous people down." The caller had actually "been on the phone when the CRO heard numerous people coughing before the phone went dead." The job sounded pretty legit.

My partner and I staged a block away from the scene. The fire department pulled right up to the subway entrance, shortly followed by an EMS Hazmat unit! As we waited to see who would pass out by the subway opening or not come back up, we were joined by EMS Cpt. Jo Ann Kovac. After the incident, she came over to my partner and I.

"Jim, would you take a walk with me over to the battalion commander?"

There was a pause, then, "He won't talk to a female."

Let's see the exploits of Engine 082.
Date: February 4, 2001
Call Type: Unconscious
Address: 1488 Hoe Ave. (Church)
Assign: Engine 082
12:36:38 PD Comp (T61) Fm Fl Mn-AT
Church-CB-Aided 28Y/O OPR 2291 (8643)
12:36:58 Entry (*643) FCS F28 UNC

156

12:36:58 Final Ack Cent to PD (8643)
12:36:58 Fire Sent (8643) Call sent to Fire
12:37:03 Fire Ack 04Feb 0112352301035273
12:37:15 FIRE ASSIGNED 04Feb01123537 E082 (Engine 082)
12:37:26 Assign (0899) 26W2 (Paramedics)
12:37:29 Enroute (2831) 26W2
12:40:43 Supplement-PD (D11A) 042E Assigned
12:41:00 FIRE ON SCENE 04Feb01123922 E082 (Engine 082)
12:42:15 On scene (2831) 26W2
12:42:48 Fire Clear 04 Feb01124109 E082
12:42:49 Fire Close 04 Feb 01124110

According to this, we have a female unconscious in a church. It would appear that Engine 082 was on the scene awaiting our arrival for over a minute. Remember, heart and brain cells die in four to six minutes.

As we unloaded our equipment, one gentleman from the church asked if we needed help or wanted cars moved. He also looked up the block and asked, "Is that fire truck coming here also?"

"No sir," my partner answered. We proceeded to the patient. Engine 82 was never at the predominately black church in the South Bronx.

The truth is sad and evident to those of us who serve ghetto communities. These firemen do not want to do the job for which they've been paid and tasked. They can hop on their trucks, get credit for the calls, and get the extra taxpayers' money—and not give a shit about the people who are paying for a service. The people deserve better.

This would never happen in Midtown Manhattan, where there are lawyers, cameras, and wealthy, influential residents. This was the secret learned by the crews concerning going from five-men engines to four.

Rumor had it that the firefighters' union freaked because up to that point there were five people on an engine, four cameramen, and one firefighter. The union, realizing how the Fire God ran the department, was petrified the one guy to be knocked off the truck would be the lone firefighter!

These stories are quite different from the one painted in the Report from Engine Company 82 by firefighter Dennis Smith. Mr. Smith's writings reflect well upon those who truly serve the public and it is my belief there are honorable, hardworking men. But even Mr. Smith would agree that there has been a cancerous growth of epidemic proportions that has been allowed to fester. Only now are its fruits starting to surface.

If allowed to continue, it will eventually implode the image of the job he, heroes like firefighter-academy instructor Jim Myerjack, who changed consciousness (died) from cancer, and firefighter Kevin C. Kane (Ladder 110, and a former EMT, who paid the ultimate price by having his gear grotesquely melted to his body while searching for squatters in an abandoned building). Or current heroes—men of conscience like Lt. Kevin Pfeifer (Engine 33), a former Bellevue EMS paramedic, my cousin Jerry Schrang (Rescue 3), and the crew of Engine One, and Squad 61—who all love the job and the public they serve. These are the real "Bravest," and not the majority.

Regarding the politicians' fraudulent claims that CFRD Program was working, Res Ipsa Loquitor, the facts speak for themselves.

To have the First Responder Program work, we need three basic things: a crew that gets to the job and a crew on the scene that knows what to do and does it correctly.

The fire trucks are either not getting to the scene, not going to the scene, or when there, just sitting on their asses outside the job. Doesn't this constitute fraud?

In the South Bronx, the majority of engine companies I have seen have neither the professional expertise nor personal character of the crews on Engine One in Manhattan, and that is pathetic. But the problem within the firehouse has been aided and abetted by a mayor who believes he is above the law.

Mayoral wannabes supported the lawsuit by our union (2507). The lawsuit found that Mayor Giuliani circumvented the city charter requirements when he and his poster child, the fire commissioner, brought in for-profit ambulance service MetroCare. Mark Green even acknowledged the "law and order" mayor circumvented the law.

Is it just me? Or do you think there is a case of corruption here? First, a CFR Program that is not working, and then instead of funding its own FDEMS units, it goes to a Giuliani crony who has contributed a lot of money to his election. When something looks like shit, smells like shit, and, well, I'll leave the tasting up to the fire commissioner, EMS command, and mayor since a load of shit comes out of their mouths.

Concerning the fire commissioner, he seemed to think he and Chief Peter J. Ganci Jr. (Chief of Department) had the knowledge to run EMS.

If, perchance, sound fiscal management is required for cost effectiveness, why have firemen delivering checks when the EMT Borough Supply Coordinator is only allowed to pick up stationery at 9 Metro Tech Headquarters? Is it true the fire department hired an outside firm to deliver mail? If so, how costly was that deal? Why has more than one fireman been on light duty for periods of up to ten years and EMS crews are sent to the unemployment line after eighteen months? How is management justified, by having FDNY fire lieutenants who make about $62,000 a year handing out belts and hats in the Quarter Master Shop?

Or the fire captain making $90,000 a year paid watching the lieutenants?

Wouldn't it be fiscally prudent to place civilians in these cushy jobs? Do any of these geniuses have a clue that three people could be hired for the price of one $90,000-a-year fire captain? Think how much good could really be done for three people on welfare who don't want to be there.

Wouldn't this help the unemployed of New York, especially single mothers, and get the trained, experienced members back fighting fires and teaching the probees? Out of a reported 11,000 firefighters, how many are actually in the firehouse? If an EMT or paramedic can't do our jobs, we are fired. Handing out shoes, crappy ones at that, or moving furniture sure sounds outside of a firefighter's job description, especially if the furniture isn't burning.

Or let's look at the new "Fire Ego Shop" located on Fifth Avenue in Manhattan. Why is a firefighter there, collecting a paycheck talking to tourists and selling FDNY baseball hats and sweatshirts instead of fighting fires? I would like to see an investigation determine the number of firefighters "hidden" in cushy details such as BHS, Information and Computer Services, Support Facilities, and the like. Also, *where is all this money going?* But more on that later, and I'm sick of hearing "fire prevention programs" as the answer. If that was the truth, there would never be another fire in New York City.

Still, EMS Command would not be outdone by FD in ineptness, or putting their futures ahead of either the Street Saints or the public. In February of 1998, the paramedic units received Atropine and 2Pam kits for a chemical attack. Next they were placed in the trunks of EMS chiefs' cars as if they could be counted on to back us up in an emergency.

Finally, and much later, the Basic units were issued Atropine and 2Pam kits. The federal government had informed us, New York City would get hit it. The first bombing of the World Trade Center had been a wakeup call for the federal government, but not for our gods. With the distribution of the kits, we requested gas masks. The request fell on deaf ears in the Medical Director's Office. Doctors jockeyed for position, cutting each other's throats to appear as the golden choice to the Fire God.

To quell any fear, Chief Gabrielle came to our station to disclose that Dr. Darrio Gonzales had set up the plan for such an incident and that we, the EMS crews, would be in the "Cold Zone." This came from a doctor who had never seen combat. We learned some information from medical students entering the EMS fellowship program. They told us of his derogatory remarks about the paramedics. This was from a man who went out to the federal building explosion, never recovered a body, but reportedly was traumatically affected by what he saw.

Evidently, his experience didn't translate into common sense, compassion or concern for EMS crews within his responsibility. He didn't read The Art of War by Sun Tzu or realize that combat is fluid in nature, not static like firehouse mentality.

Instead, he had a dog and pony show at Bellevue, the ultimate ground zero. The EMS instructors told us the truth. It was a ploy to appease us and the casualties would be high. In fact, the gods already accepted massive EMS losses, which was totally unacceptable to combat veterans like paramedic Lou Cook and myself.

An EMT asked the chief, "What happens if we are at ground zero, in a cold zone, and the wind shifts?"

"You'll be dead," he said in a cold, unemotional voice. When we asked again about protective masks, we were told none would be coming.

From the chemical attack in Japan, they had learned about off gassing and put it to good use. The chiefs reportedly had a computer model to show how many trips an unprotected EMT could make to the hospital, ambulance loaded with casualties, before he was overcome by the off gases! At this point it was hard to decide who the bigger asshole was, the Medical Director or the chief for thinking anyone in their right mind would respond in. Between the two of them they couldn't lead a blind deaf mute to an over ripe shithouse as far as I was concerned. There was one thing I was deadly sure of and that was that neither was worth a pimple on the worst EMT's ass. Oh, as a side note Eddie Gabrielle in 2006 was hired by Walt Disney. Hey, hey credit where credit is due, the man's career was spent in the Enchanted Forest of EMS where delusion, I mean fantasy rules.

After much research, Lou Cook and I got the specs for the gas masks and filters we wanted and the search was on. I went to Samgong Industrial Company in Seoul, Korea. Their GM (Gas Mask)-148K with K-1 canister was just the item we needed. Then I adapted an American Chemical Biological hood. Numerous delays followed.

Chief Robert McCracken, in charge of the EMS Bureau, met with us on August 13, 1998 at Battalion Eight, Kips Bay Station in Bellevue. The meeting had been put off several times because the chief had to attend local community board meetings, showing where his priority was once again.

Below is an excerpt of a letter I sent Chief Robert McCracken on August 17, 1998. It says a lot about the mentality of the civilian chiefs of EMS as well as the Fire God.

". . . I'm bringing to your attention that the lackluster program which paramedics were given, as directed by Dr. Gonzales to satisfy a federal mandate, was not in compliance with federal guidelines, nor did it demonstrate any sound combat logic. To reiterate, we have been told that Fire Suppression, (Firemen) as well as our ERS (Emergency Response Squad, glorified HazTac) crews will be in protective gear. We (EMTs and Paramedics) will be in the Warm Zone. We will not be wearing protective gear or have escape hoods available because Dr. Gonzales has 'Drawn the Circles.'

The thinking is non-combat wishful thinking by the politically correct. It will deplete our resources and increase causalities of our EMS crews. It will make nil our ability to protect the Fire Suppression and ERS Teams in the Hot Zone or serve the public. Instead it will aid and serve said terrorists in their attempt to inflict maximum casualties with minimum loss to their side. This mentality, is also in direct violation of Janes Chem-Bio Handbook. Endorsed by Mayor Rudolph Guiliani, Howard Safir, Commissioner NYPD, Jerome Hauer, Director, Mayors Office of Emergency Management and Thomas Von Essen, Commissioner, NYFD, as our guidelines for such terrorist attack. It is a doctrine supported by our military, as they are the supporting co-authors.

I explained why I had decided on the GM-148K with K-1 canister with the adaptation of the chemical bio hood standard with the United States Army. The result of this letter was interesting.

Deputy Chief Randy Hirth had asked me about the masks, but he never gave me a hard time about them. I have worked several MCIs (mass casualty incidents) with him and his aide, Grace Cacciola. I honestly cannot think of a single time I had a problem with the way either one conducted an operation. He was always supportive of his people. All he required was we do our jobs.

This was not the case of Division Commander Pedro Carrasquillo. During my meeting with Chief McCracken, I voiced my belief that Division Commander Carrasquillo had repeatedly demonstrated his inability to be effective and to appreciate that Manhattan was target-rich for a terrorist strike. He demonstrated inability to logically answer why EMS medic units were changed at a whim or why it appeared the voluntary units got the better hours. He had an inept statement: "You are assigned a tour." That was not an answer.

After my meeting with Chief McCracken, I had another shipment of masks on the way, since more people wanted to buy them. At Bellevue, the chief asked me, "By whose authority are you carrying that? Who knows about this? Who is sanctioning this? Is the union aware of this?"

Paramedic Tom Reynolds laughed as I said, "Let's see how long it takes before he starts trouble."

One week later, paramedic Lou Cook was summoned downtown and grilled about the masks. Then Chief Carrasquillo called the desk at Bellevue. Lieutenant Jo Ann Kovac received the call. The chief was ordering her to tell everyone, "Masks were not to be on the units, whether they were personal safety items or not. They were not issued by FD."

Then Lieutenant Kovac informed him, "Chief, if you are still standing after this is over, you can write me up." He went ballistic.

"How many masks do you have?"

"I always carry one."

"Expect a call from Captain Charlie Wells ERS (Emergency Response Squad)."

That evening, Captain Phil Para saw me in the emergency room at Bellevue. "Oh, so you are the guy selling these?" As if he didn't know. He is down at Station Eleven with the Borough Office (the Enchanted Forest) where Chief Carrasquillo resides.

"I think I'll get one. Can I see yours?" A discussion followed and I gave him the information. He knew the date of the next shipment, country of origin, and the like. I saw it all coming and was letting it happen, because as usual I was one step ahead of these amateurs. Dear old Pedro and the rest of the gang were spending a lot of energy to ensure our people *weren't protected*. If half of this energy was expended ensuring the safety of EMTs and paramedics, we would stand a fighting chance. But that was not EMS supervision. Whatever their move, I knew I could and would beat it.

As expected, they made their move. Or was it coincidence again? On April 23, 1998, a week after my little talk with Captain Para, I received a phone call from a customs agent at JFK International Airport. He told me, "You have to come over and sign a form so the shipment can be released."

"Any problem?" I asked.

"Oh no! You need to sign a form and you'll have your items."

I went over in my little fire department superman outfit and took them by surprise. I cordially mixed in and walked through the so-called security. I stood in front of the desk as the agent spoke on the phone. I waited for him to hang up. I introduced myself and actually startled him.

"How did you get through security?" he demanded.

"By my good looks."

When he had regained his composure, I asked about the form and I took out my pen. I realized there was more to the game.

"Please wait in this office and I'll be there in a moment."

I found myself in an interrogation room. I looked around and waited for the next act. Three agents interrogated me. They all left a lot to be desired. I asked how these items were flagged and was told, "By the item name, gas masks."

"Cool," I said, asking, "How come my other shipment wasn't flagged?"

"The quantity of this shipment." That's funny because this was a smaller shipment.

"Who dropped the quarter? Was it Chief Carrasquillo? He is the only one giving me a hard time."

These amateurs never even asked, "Who?" This blew right over him, as I confirmed what I already knew. Next they wanted to see the paperwork and my identification. They ran a computer search on me, and it showed I was clean. They even went over the costs, and it demonstrated I was not making a profit. They were having a bad day. Finally, they asked whom I worked for. I stated Captain Mark Stone. If these wannabe interrogators wanted to be like the real ones, they would have come back at me once I said Captain Mark Stone's name. The least they could have asked, "But who is Chief Carrasquillo? I thought he was your boss."

I received more information from them by their sloppy non-professional approach than they ever got from me. After I said their actions were illegal, I was released. They could find nothing, since there was nothing to find. Still, I stayed one step ahead of them. I called the station, since I had taken the day without pay, and spoke to Captain Stone. I told him to expect a phone call from customs. Sure enough, the next day when I got to work, he told me they called. They asked if I worked for him and if he knew anything about the masks.

"Sure I do. We are all waiting for them."

That was it. I contacted a licensed customs house broker and I delivered the shipment several days later. By the way, Captain Para never ordered a mask.

On April 26, 1998, Lieutenant Charlie Frazier told paramedic Lou Cook that "if someone falls wearing the masks they will be denied LODI (Line of Duty Injury)." This was a really intelligent statement, since the only reason the crew _would_ wear them was if their lives were threatened by a chemical or biological attack. His next statement told me why the good chief was trying to stop me. Lieutenant Frazier stated, "Fire is upset because the masks are unfitted and the crews untrained." Hello... we would not be going through this if EMS and fire were concerned for our safety. On April 29, 1998, I made the delivery to the crews at Bellevue and yes, Lieutenant Charlie Frazier became an EMS captain.

Captain Charlie Wells of ERS mysteriously showed up to talk to me about the masks. He told me of the great job he'd heard I had done in Bosnia. Old news, but I guess he figured it was a way of playing to my ego.

When he finally got around to the masks he told me, "NYC has brought masks for EMS already." Gee if this were true where were they?

"Escape masks are for EMS, _not masks_ that let you stay and survive in a hostile environment. EMS will be in a Cold Zone. These (escape masks) won't be worn until _my_ ERS units tell you to 'Don and escape' since the Cold Zone is now Warm. Besides, Fire wants to know, 'Who the hell is Schrang?'" Yeah like I'm going to wait until this rum-dumb asshole who has a more colorful history than a decorated fuckin Christmas tree comes out of the 'hot zone' to say, "Don and Escape! You're fuckin contaminated!" Yeah right I thought looking at him with a blank poker face.

He continued, "I want a mask so I can tear it apart to find its weakness, so _you_ don't get into trouble."

What a buddy! To reiterate with his colorful background, what more could I ask for in my corner?

"I called Chief Carrasquillo and told him they were not allowed on the unit."

This final point was really interesting. I never did, nor ever will, trust Charlie Wells. I did not ask about the good chief and his phone call to the station. Since when does a captain tell a chief in the form of an order what can or can't be done? Finally, I told the good captain I would be willing to sit in a chamber with him. He could wear his escape mask he claimed the city already bought, and I'd wear the GM-148K with K-1 canister. "I'll sit in there for not one hour, but twenty-four hours, then walk out and piss in your pocket." I believed in *my* equipment that much. I didn't tell him I had already given a mask with a canister to Chief McCracken, who delivered it to the Fire God's Chief Steven King, NYC Fire Safety at 9 Metro Tech. Soon Hack Hong, the representative from Samgong Industrial Co. Ltd. in South Korea, also contacted Chief King. The letter went out on August 22, 1998.

Since he wasn't up to the challenge I informed the good captain that in the military, something he knows nothing about, the only form-fitted masks, so to speak, are flight crew masks. I know, since aside from being an army paratrooper, I also flew with the Air Force Reserve. Nor does the fire department fit their Scott masks. His answer was, "Well, if you have a strange face." Side note here: Yes gentle reader this genius became an EMS Chief but you'll read more about him on 9-11-'01.

Concerning training, I took each person and explained the care and use of the mask and filter. In combat, like in a terrorist strike, you cannot afford to lose resources, especially foolishly. Even with escape masks, the EMTs and paramedics would become casualties. The public would lose medical crews, already a scarce resource.

I brought up immunizations. The military has them. Why not EMS? Do you know how many units in Queens respond to a "sick" on a plane landing from an international flight? I was informed that Dr. Gonzales was against it.

167

In closing, I will extract the final paragraph of my letter to Chief McCracken.

"Finally, there is NO CONFIDENCE at street level for EMS Management, or ERS after what they did to us at Gramercy Park."(Gramercy Park is located South of Bellevue Hospital. A giant steam pipe created a massive explosion killing several people. Being the second bus on the scene, I aided two workers who were burned to death. Our SOD, later ERS, with the fire department knew in the first fifteen minutes there was a massive asbestos release.

They never said a word to us. Several months later we read the fire department was suing for the loss of contaminated equipment, clothing etc. Know what EMS Management did? They ordered us to bring in our clothes. They then decontaminated the buses, the same ones that so many people had been transported in long after the incident.)

I continued, "That is why to the person, each EMT and paramedic, has refused to follow the order of Chief Carrasquello not to carry the GM148K on their units as 'personal safety items.'"

If a picture is worth a thousand words, I have two photos that were taken and sent worldwide. On August 8, 2000, a rush-hour bomb exploded in a busy walkway in Moscow. As our Russian EMS brothers retrieved the wounded and dead, they wore gas masks and gloves. The other photo appeared in the New York Times, on September 1, 2000. It shows construction workers entering a fire department decontamination truck to be washed down after being exposed to asbestos. The firemen were at the door, ready for the workers. The firemen donned gas masks and protective clothing. Next to the yellow line stood an EMS EMT, in short sleeve shirt, wearing no gloves, but worse, no mask. Captain Mark Stone ran the operation. You be the judge of which EMS System is working toward being ready.

Our people were still unprotected. The city never bought the escape masks, or any other claimed by Captain Wells. There was talk of refurbishing the Vietnam-era masks and storing them at a central location for the transit police.

That sure as hell makes a lot of sense. I got back the test mask from Chief King. He never found anything wrong with it.

The only problem here lies with the fire gods and civilian gods of EMS. These politically correct ass wipes do not understand that the United States of America is at war. Unless we have a Pearl Harbor with fuckin Fundamentalist Muslims riding surfboards through the front door, our managers will not recognize what is happening. New York City, thanks to the ineptness that festers within both the fire and EMS commands, has placed civilians at great risk. I feared for our EMS crews.

FDNY keeps up the image at all costs, including the truth... On the cover of one edition of Fire Works was the headline, "Commissioner's Message Being a Real Boss Means Making the Tough Decisions." In the article the commissioner proudly proclaimed giving pensions to his brothers, after they lied and falsified documents.

I have a suggestion. Instead of he and his cronies pretending to be bosses and making "hard decisions," perhaps he and his brothers should try to be men and tell the truth. Only then can they become bosses who can make "tough decisions." The public deserves it. Firefighters of honor, as the one aforementioned, deserve it. And we, EMS people, demand it.

The Fire God and his little flamer civilian gods, EMS civilian chiefs, are inept, greedy, egotistical, hypercritical, and downright liars. They have decimated the EMS Street Saints of Compassion. We are enraged that the job we loved was destroyed by the likes of Mr. Von Essen and his dimwitted cronies.

I will say this in their defense. They saw a great thing and took it. To the victor go the spoils. Even to this day, the civilian EMS chiefs have made it all possible, along with this book. It was *they* who ruled by fear and intimidation. It was *they* who were spineless and ball-less, singing the praises of the Fire God in front of the city council. It was *they* who wanted us moved into facilities the Fire God deemed uninhabitable. It was *they* who were more concerned about the Fire God's ego than our safety on the gas mask issue. It was *they* who rode the coattails of every union contract, looking for more. It goes on and on. The mayor rewarded the fire department with a golden lamb because he knew the chiefs would toe the line. But then people without spine always do. These are the real culprits.

I have always believed what goes around, comes around. It would not surprise me to hear that the EMS civilian chiefs' titles were changed to "unit managers." Then they could be reduced at any time and a fire department battalion chief could take over. I for one feel this would make total sense and accomplish something I've wanted all along—to get rid of these people.

The fire department should take the most experienced and capable EMS captains, of the caliber of Debbie Monty, Carl Tramontana, Andy Werner, Jerrold Gelbard and place them in the borough chiefs' slots. They should be captains with substantial salary increases. They in turn would answer to the fire department battalion chief.

The other EMS captains, with their long, colorful histories, would be dumped. Several captains may need work, like Werner, but they are more than capable of being molded into true leaders by stronger peers. But this would, could only happen if FDNY had vision and could see beyond their ego. Currently, these captains are wasting away and the fire department is throwing away needed talent. But what else is new? I really do not see a truly beneficial mentoring peer group scenario for these officers or even EMS. This, I reiterate, is the result of the blossoming of destruction within the parent organization. Instead of visionaries within the FDNY, you have dysfunctional rum buddies whose ineptness is flaunted by their need to employ lies and draconian rules.

FDNY prides itself on being the Bravest, but they will never, ever be the smartest.

Yet the Follies continue. In the New York of July 13, 2001, there was a story headlined, "Fire Chief in Drug Bust." According to the article, "Robert Gleason, forty-three, a twenty-three-year veteran of the fire department assigned to Battalion Thirty-seven in Brooklyn, was pulled over on the service road of the Van Wyck Expressway near One Hundred Ninth Avenue on his way home from work. When the cops asked Gleason to take his hands out of his pockets, he allegedly tried to stuff a bag of pot in his pants. He also tried to discard the painkillers, Vicodin and Oxycontin. Gleason was charged with possession of marijuana and a controlled substance. The FDNY had no immediate comment."

I wondered how the spin team in the FDNY public relations section was going to overcome this. How long would it take them to play the hearts-and-roses press game? Let's look at what appeared the next day in the Daily News, dated July 24, 2001:

"A veteran fire department battalion chief was held on $100,000 bail yesterday after Queens prosecutors charged him with possessing the hot designer drug Oxycontin. Queens Criminal Court Judge Suzanne Melendez set the high bail and announced, 'I'm not going to release him.'

"Prosecutors had requested $500,000 bail, citing the seriousness of the case. Melendez ignored a plea by Gleason's lawyer, James Mochella, to release the battalion chief to a detoxification bed in Flushing Hospital Medical Center."

Here's what the cops actually found. Fifty or more pills. Eight were Oxycontin tablets and the remainder were Vicodin, pain killers. Cops also found eighteen empty narcotic prescription bottles, and a small amount of marijuana. The prosecutors described Oxycontin as a synthetic opiate that creates a powerful addiction. Mochella said, "It's going to become clear that Chief Gleason may have substance abuse problems from a chronic injury sustained on the job while fighting a fire in the summer of 2000."

Give me a break. He was coming from work. If he was on drugs at work, that's illegal. It would put the crews, as well as the public, in danger.

For someone who reportedly "*may* have a problem" due to a fire over a year ago, I ask two questions. First, when was the last time anyone has seen a NYFD, oh I'm sorry, that's FDNY. Please note in NYPD, New York comes first. In NYEMS, New York comes first. In NYDS, New York comes before dept. of Sanitation. Only in the ego driven fire department does Fire Department come *before* New York folks. But back to the story here. When has anyone seen an FDNY battalion chief carry more than his radio? I sure as hell haven't.

Next, if he was hurt and medicated, BHS should have it documented. How did he pass his yearly physicals? If it was documented, what the hell was he doing on the job where peoples' lives are at stake? Finally, injury or not, who gave him the drugs and marijuana? Last I heard, marijuana is illegal.

You'd think the guy would be fired and have to forfeit pay. But remember, spin city FDNY public relations has helped place others on disability pensions for far less. Perhaps the department will send him to the local "farm" where they send their alcoholic brothers to dry out. Yeah, these are the places that DOI claim they have no information on...

Did you know FDNY "Calendars of Heroes" have brought in over $250,000 since first published in 1996? So where's the money going? Why the Fire Safety Education Fund of course...

Seven
The Making of New Legends

James Patrick "Bubba" Fallar is a short, balding, swashbuckling munchkin. He is one of those very special people in EMS of whom legends are made, not only in his mind. Bubba will always be known, not so much for his work as a medic, but for his snoring and famous sayings.

Don't misunderstand he's a good medic, when you can get him awake, as all who have had the pleasure of working with him know.

Throughout history, we have had famous sayings in America like, "Remember the Alamo." But we shall never forget, James Patrick "Bubba" Fallar's Hindenburg Twelve, or his famous, "Disregard me. Get to the patient!"

Bubba and I first met one dark chaotic evening at a shooting on a Harlem street corner.

My partner and friend, paramedic Harvey Feintuch, and I, Stress Free 10Z, were on the Central frequency when we were assigned the "Shot." Initially we idled in our lair under the Central Park trees, then exited the shadow of the trees at the north end of the park picking up speed, entering Harlem. Gaining velocity, I looked North on Lenox Avenue and saw the lights of multiple Harlem EMS units converging on our job!

We were never second to anyone so I engaged the dilithium crystals as Harvey and I went ballistic warp factor five.

Bubba, a new paramedic, was driving with this loser lieutenant from Harlem. As they responded, another Harlem medic unit, 18 Young, launched dramatically from their resting nest on a softly lit side-street. Aboard were EMS legends paramedics Thomas Giorgi, a Vietnam veteran, and Richard Stein, both friends and Richie a hero of the genocide in Bosnia. Both of these legends looked to the south and realized the darting lights belonged to Stress Free. The game was on. They literally blew by the patrol boss's vehicle, cutting sharply in front of him to avoid a stopped vehicle. As the rear of their ambulance filled the windshield of the unsuspecting officer, he screamed. The officer hit the brakes of the command vehicle, recovering at the last minute as the rear end fishtailed, nearly hitting a parked car.

Bouncing around inside, sliding across the seat, Bubba frantically grasped the buckle and attached his seatbelt in the careening vehicle. His eyes widened incredibly, as he focused on the swerving 18 Young in front of his windshield. Just as quickly as the unit pulled away from the rattled lieutenant's command vehicle, Bubba saw the lights to the south moving even faster and wondered," Who are those guys?" He was focused on the race and could feel the tension rising, as he ignored the curses coming from the pale EMT lieutenant driving.

The officer vocalized what Bubba had been wondering, "Fuckin' paramedics! I wonder who those crazy bastards are?"

I looked up Lenox Avenue and saw traffic sitting at a red light in front of us. I knew 18 Young was gaining ground to take full advantage of the tactical situation and would beat us.

"Hang on, Harvey," I said in calm and reassuring tone, as Stress Free banked, jumped, and accelerated across the concrete island, moving into the oncoming traffic lane with a bounce. All the while, we picked up speed and gained ground. Swerving between cars, 18 Young was losing ground and kinetic energy.

The man "shot" was sitting against the wall on the northwest corner of Lenox Avenue. I caught the wounded man's eyes fill with terror as Stress Free jumped the curb and headed straight for him. A cloud of blue smoke engulfed the vehicle as I locked up the brakes. We came to a jolting stop, which would make any carrier-qualified jet pilot proud. I yelled Harvey, "Run to the patient. I'll get the equipment."

"What? I'll get the equipment," he said. Harvey knew I was the faster runner, but didn't want to admit it.

Out of the corner of my eye I saw Tommy jumping from his moving vehicle. I bailed out and sprinted toward the patient. I beat Tommy by about four steps, touched the patient on the shoulder, and said, "Ah ha, beat you."

Tommy was laughing as he said, "Shit, it was close."

As we checked the patient, Richie and Harvey approached with the stretcher and equipment.

The blond-headed lieutenant, I think his first or perhaps last name was Gregg, came up and commanded dramatically, "Schrang, we only need one medic unit on the scene. Get out of here, now!"

I felt the love. Such a command decision said so forcefully by this twit deserved an answer.

"Fuck off. We… the paramedics, not you, will decide who is needed here."

Tom shook his head in agreement, laughing as Harvey and Richie evaluated the patient.

"Mind if we take the job?" he asked.

"Hell, its okay with me, if it's okay with Harvey."

Harvey had no complaint, so they loaded the patient onto the long board and further evaluated him.

The police pulled up as Harvey, Richie, and Tommy worked on the man. I heard more sirens. There was a chase in progress one block over, on Adam Clayton Powell Jr. Boulevard. Some guys had robbed a car and were being chased by three police cars. The robbers made the mistake of turning down our block, heading toward the cops. Talk about a bad night.

Hurdling down the street, heading east, they swerved in panic, trying to pass the car in front of them sideswiping some cars and sending garbage cans flying like exploding missiles high into the air as civilians and cops screamed seeking cover. A lone, black female was in the car in front of them, the only thing between them and freedom. Suddenly over the screams, wailing sirens, and crashing metal, cops in the chase cars, lights flashing, yelled over the PA, "Stop that car!"

The sound echoed down the block, reverberating through the concrete canyon.

The cops with us drew their guns and jumped into the street in front of the woman's car, screaming for her to stop! Locking up the brakes, trying to avoid hitting the officers, she stopped, petrified at the sight of the guns. Suddenly the wailing sirens were shattered by a thunderous explosion and blinding flash of light. The perps' car, accelerating to escape, smashed into the rear of her car at a tremendous rate of speed.

One moment she was stopped, with officers' guns pointing at her. The next, in a split second, she was rapidly catapulted forward, bending the steering wheel and column with her chest, then roughly snapped backward with such violence the seat snapped its steel connections collapsing under horrific "g" load.

She could see the officers diving for cover as her car, totally out of control, hurtled several feet off the ground, smashing into a parked police car and coming to a bone-jarring halt.

The cops were screaming, "Shots fired!"

But the sound and flash came from the impact of metal, exploding glass, and deploying airbag in the perp's car.

Harvey, Tommy, and Richie did a low crawl with their patient. Figuring the perps came back to finish the job on this guy, all three medics opted to risk their lives for this unknown person. They were determined to get him to safety, not realizing they weren't under fire.

The cloud of dark blue and gray smoke enveloped the scene, burning my eyes and lungs as I ran to the woman's car. Needless to say, Lieutenant Twit was nowhere to be found, but I did find Bubba. He was hunched down and moving away from the scene as fast as his feet would carry him.

As he shot by, I grabbed him by his belt, so that his legs were moving but not going anywhere.

"Where the hell do you think you're going?" I asked, as I was trying to see where my three friends were. The screaming and general noise was deafening. I didn't give him a chance to speak.

"You! Stay with this woman. Understand?" I thundered.

"Yes sir," came the meek reply.

I walked through the smoke, observing the cops slam-dunk the perps on the hood of the stolen car, as they still violently resisted arrest. These idiots were real losers. I found my three friends behind 18 Young's ambulance about to load the patient, and I assisted with the lift.

As Harvey and I walked over to Bubba, I saw the twit lieutenant, white supervisor helmet on, directing a Basic unit to the crumbled car and woman. After the woman was loaded into the Basic unit, Harvey hopped onboard to work on her. I walked back to Stress Free and headed toward Harlem Hospital.

This was my first meeting with a very new, extremely diaphoretic Bubba, but luckily not my last. Later, back at the Harlem station, he told the crews when asked about the night he worked with "General Patton."

Unlike firemen who sleep in warm firehouses, with kitchens, weight and cable TV rooms we sit in ambulances twenty-four seven. Unless you are a nocturnal owl, the biggest battle one faces on these torturous tours, aside from cramping, is staying awake.

Some of us would bring reading material until the words became unreadable because of closing eye lids. Thus any distraction, especially the practical joke type, was welcome relief in assisting to keep us awake. One night, Bubba and I were working a midnight tour. Except for Bubba's tumultuous snoring, it was a quiet evening, as I pulled out of the garage at Bellevue. Bubba had curled up in the seat with his pillow supporting his head and a blanket on his lap. He went right off to sleep, all warm and cuddly.

I pulled up to Sym's Deli at Thirty-fourth Street and Lexington Avenue. Reaching over, I keyed up the mike on the radio and placed it next to Bubba's snoring lips. His snores made NASA's wind test tunnel sound like a gentle breeze.

It didn't take long before the central dispatcher begged for mercy and units who knew him yelled his name over the radio. I giggled. His eyes shot open. Startled, disoriented, he yelled, "Hey! What the . . ." This sealed his fate. Now even the central dispatcher knew what Irishman owned that deafening snore.

After getting our food, we headed down the block making what I called "Bubba's Slut Run." He enjoyed watching the ladies of the night sell their wares.

Pulling over to Lexington Avenue and Twenty-eighth Street to have our meal. This was the beginning of the vibrant Indian district. I smiled, remembering the ambrosia of the 'Curry In A Hurry' restaurant located on Lexington Avenue I passed going to work. Further south was the Pakistani area of town. Because of bloody encounters precipitated by historical hatred, even their parades had to be separated and monitored closely by the police. If asked my personal opinion based on experience, it was that the Indian population had always demonstrated an inner strength and respectful obedience to law, whereas the Pakistanis were more the wild cards, only cooperating if it was to their advantage, whether talking about the law, respect for others, or even driving cabs.

As we sat, two cars stopped at the light. Once the light turned green, the limousine in the extreme left lane made a sharp, unexpected right turn, tearing off the front bumper of the car in the right lane that was going straight. The owner of the damaged car got out and yelled at the other driver. The limo emptied of five gentlemen from Pakistan. It was five to one. The lone driver, looking like a dorky Alfred E. Newman, was in over his head. Outnumbered and unable to beat his way out of this mess, he hollered for the police, like a person lacking testosterone.

Hearing the high-pitched shriek and observing the miscarriage of justice, Officer Bubba responded. The cuddly blanket was cast aside in determined fashion, as he dramatically threw open the bus door. Gently letting himself down to the ground, pulling up the belt on his pants, under his pot belly, Bubba waddled into the fray. The whining, ear-pop-ping, nauseating shrill was drawing a lot of attention from the ladies, and prospective customers. Still, Bubba tenaciously advanced, a true beacon of hope.

After a chuckle, I had another sip of coffee, took off my glasses, and with a sigh, placed them on the dash. Getting out, I stretched, locked the unit, and moseyed on down the block. I observed Officer Bubba, mag-light in hand, trying to calm and separate the verbal combatants. He wasn't having much success, especially since most were taller than him.

Come to think of it, most people are taller than him.

Since the Pakistanis were surrounding my little buddy, I decided to assist him in his good deed for the night. Looking at one Pakistani, who was running his mouth too close to Bubba, "Hey, just back up and be cool, okay?" I said in a monotone voice, keying up my radio. "Stress Free to Central," I went on while watching this guy in front of me.

"Central to Stress Free."

"Location: Lexington and Twenty-eighth Street. We need a sector for an accident." Hearing this, the guy started to get in my face.

"Are you guys okay?" asked the dispatcher.

"Central, it's getting a little nasty here," I said in a calm, almost bored voice, yet realizing where this was going. The dispatcher heard the screams as the Pakistanis, feeling power in numbers, closed in, tightening the circle on Bubba and me. By the way, Alfred E. Newman had found refuge across the street, a typical spectator. We were now being shoved, so I gently nudged the big mouth away from me.

One of the 'ladies' walked over.

"Listen, why don't you leave the paramedics alone? They're only trying to help."

"Shut up, bitch!" the Paki yelled.

"Hey, take it easy on the lady," Bubba responded. Oh, that fighting Irish spirit!

"You can't do anything. You're not a police officer," the Pakistani defiantly yelled, inciting the fury in the others. This was developing into a bad, very bad B movie.

"I'm telling you to back up," I said with more force.

"Why, because you're an American?" he asked, shoving more forcefully.

I don't like being told what to do and the final straw for me was badmouthing America. These third-world, subhuman life forms made it clear they were only here to make money and did not have to pay attention to our laws. They'd make their money and leave.

On one previous occasion I was informed by another cabbie of same national origin, "I don't have to obey your laws. I'm here for the money!"

These dirt bag Pakistanis were a disgrace to the other millions of good, hardworking immigrants who come here, busting their asses for years, working in sweatshops at low wages and long hours. These people contribute and are the foundation of the America I know and love. I'll be the first to say there is a lot wrong here, but it is still the best game in town. But like my grandparents, they enrich this country with their culture, respect for the law, and hard work. But this was not the case with these guys.

"No, not because I'm an American. Because I'm a fuckin' American!"

I paused. To ensure he got the point, I stood on his sandaled foot, looking into his now extremely pain- and tear-filled eyes. To add an exclamation point, I dug my finger deep in his puny chest, then after a pause continued, "Asshole!"

The crowd went wild. Out of the corner of my eye, I saw another idiot's fist inbound toward me. Bubba yelled. I spun around, deflected the punch, and threw one of my own.

Bubba went on the offensive, nailing two guys with his mag-light. My return punch hit its mark, smashing into the guy's face. I followed up with a boot to his scrotal area, missing as he sidestepped and swung again. My fist crashed into his face, as he turned to run, but I followed up the block. When I caught up with him, he swung again, missing. This time my kick was on target. As he doubled over in agony I put him in a headlock, proceeding to pound him harder.

The guy was in his early twenties and bigger than me. I was almost fifty. Yet he was crying and this infuriated me even more. As I tuned him, one of the 'ladies' walked by.

"Hi," she said with a smile.

"Hi there. You be safe tonight," I said, returning the smile, as I resumed beating this crying piece of shit wearing his traditional pajamas.

EMS units had responded, as well as the police, but they were at the far end of the block. I figured the guy had enough, grabbed him by the collar, and started walking back.

Bubba, realizing I had taken off, told the crews and cops to hold the others, while he ran up the block looking for me. Running? It was running for him, but it would be half-stepping for anyone else. Bubba spotted me as I walked back into the lighted street.

A Hispanic guy with a beer stepped out of the bodega. Bubba raised the mag-light and let out a war cry, "Get the fuck away from my partner!"

He was such an awesome sight, the poor guy almost dropped his beer, as he stumbled away to avoid Officer Bubba's wrath.

Back at the corner, Bubba told a female sergeant from the Seventeenth Precinct we were assaulted.

"What are these guys, stupid?" she asked the Pakis.

"Just real assholes, Sarge," I said. She looked at me as they stood mute, licking their wounds.

"How bad is that hand of yours?"

"It's fine."

"If you want, we'll lock them up for assault."

"Do you guys want collars tonight?" I asked, realizing they were usually down on sector cars and manpower at night.

"Not really. I'm short on people. But we could give them a few tickets and hit them in their wallets. If that's good enough for you guys," she honestly queried, looking at Bubba and me.

"Yeah, that's cool," I said, glancing over and seeing the culprits trying now to shove two cops.

The sergeant saw too, "You were right," she muttered, walking over to the group. "Hey! I want your attention." One guy shoved her! Suddenly there was a flurry of fists and night sticks, the idiots stood licking their bruised bodies and deflated egos.

"You assholes will show respect to the paramedics. These guys are just like us, part of a team, our American team! Understand?"

They didn't move, but it didn't take a rocket scientist to see the depraved, foreboding and deep hatred flashing in their dark eyes.

The idiots got tickets in excess of one hundred and twenty dollars each. We all got back into our vehicles. The losers decided to take our plate number on the front of the bus.

I called the Sarge, who was inside her vehicle. She started to get out.

"Don't even, Sarge, I'll handle it." I stepped on the gas and watched the screaming idiots fly in all directions. Officer Bubba got a chuckle over the PA, "Unauthorized flight from the scene of an accident is a misdemeanor!"

"I think you did enough crime fighting for one night . . . Officer Bubba."

"You're right," he said, covering himself with his blanket, adjusting his pillow. "Call me if you need anything."

The next day "Alfred E. Newman" showed up at the garage, not to say thanks. The puke just wanted our names for his insurance company report.

You think saving lives in the big city is easy huh?

Later that night, we got a call to back up a crew responding to a "cardiac arrest." Bubba and I entered the apartment to find Karl Dykman and his full-bosomed partner giving CPR to a seventy-year-old Hispanic male.

Bubba went to the patient's head and intubated him on the first attempt. He was on a roll.

After the first round of drugs down the tube, the patient was still in that "eternal basic rhythm" asystole, better known as death. Our pace was rapid, as we tried to get some reaction from the old man's heart. I had a problem with IV insertion on the old man's arms and hands. I looked at his feet for a possible site, when Bubba said he had a good neck vein.

Sure enough, he got the IV access in the neck. Bubba ran to the phone, in view of the grieving family, and called our doctors in telemetry for more medications.

As far as I was concerned, the guy was beyond circling the drain, he was FUBAR (Fucked Up Beyond Repair) and his spirit had left the scene.

Karl whispered to me that the only reason he and his partner started working him was to console the family. I had no problem with that. The outcome would be the same, but at least the family would know we tried.

As Karl bagged the patient with the BVM, his partner did the compressions. Karl asked if she was all right. She looked as white as a ghost and complained of chest pain. What to do, you ask?

She stood up, holding on to a chair facing Bubba on the phone. The family, and now present New York's Finest, wanted to see more of her.

I looked down at the patient, who wasn't going anywhere, and removed the cardiac cables attached to his chest. Karl knew what was coming. He tried to shield his partner from the onlookers, as I approached her with the cables and new EKG pasties.

She started to open her blouse. I stood in front, blocking the view. Her watermelon-sized breasts seemed to explode from her skimpy lace bra. Karl's eyes bulged through his steaming glasses, as I grabbed a peek at the monitor, he at his partner's jutting brown nipples. The screen showed sinus tachycardia, the same a healthy person gets from working out or running to the bus.

Bubba was on the phone with the doctor, explaining we should call the arrest and pronounce the patient dead. As the doctor gave him the time, he glanced at the monitor and saw a normal rhythm, thinking it was from the dead guy.

"Jim," I heard over my shoulder.

"Chill out, Bubba," I told him, as I went back to asking the EMT more questions.

"Jim…"

"Will you be quiet, Bubba?"

"Stand by doctor, uh Jim?"

"What do you want?" I demanded stepping away from the EMT.

Bubba's eyes shot like lightning from the monitor to her erect nipples to me, then faster than light back to the EMT's melons.

After regaining his composure, putting eyes back in his head, and wiping drool off his mouth, he babbled into the phone, "Thanks, doc," and abruptly hung up.

According to Bubba, he not only intubated and got the IV going, but he alone, saved the man's life thinking the sinus-tach on the monitor was from the dead guy.

Several years ago, a big deal was made in the newspapers concerning the save rate of cardiac arrests in Washington state as opposed to New York City. The headlines screamed that you were more likely to be saved by the paramedics in Seattle than by paramedics in New York. If the media had read the report, which they didn't, they'd have seen that Seattle paramedics have tighter parameters for working an arrest and don't work certain rhythms. If CPR is not instituted within a certain time, if the medics are not on the scene in a specific time, and if you are not in one of the rhythms that their medical control doctors deem workable, you are dead. NYC EMS will work up anyone, at anytime, trying to beat the eternal clock.

The papers tried playing our paramedics against theirs and their medications against ours. The fact is, their paramedics are just as good, and just as bad, as ours. Also, there is merit to their approach, but in a world of Dan Rather personalities instead of investigative reporting you get canned useless crap stirred up for the emotionalism, nothing more, nothing less.

You might think Bubba is gullible, but not this Irish giant among clover. Nothing gets past him, well, almost nothing. One day, I typed out a form directing him to report at said time to headquarters, the CCU. I placed it in an envelope and marked it confidential in bright red letters.

At work, Bubba was given the document. As I watched, I could see the confusion and concern on his beet-red face. It was cute watching his blood pressure rise up his neck, to his ears and then face.

Upon opening it, he read the name and officer he was supposed to call, prior to reporting in. I suggested he call, which he did promptly, while the silent crews watched.

"Hello? Ah yes, this is paramedic James Fallar. Yes, James Fallar. I've been directed to call a Lieutenant Abadabadu."

"Who?" asked the party on the other end.

"Lieutenant Abadabadu."

"Please say that again?" the EMT on the other end requested.

Bubba looked disgusted.

"Say it slow, Bubba," I said, almost unable to hold a straight face.

"Lieutenant Ab-a-Dab-a-Du . . ." Without completing the sentence, he looked at me as the crews roared.

"Fuck you, Schrang," our hero said, as he slammed down the phone.

It was really great. But so is our legend.

I was not the only one to pull a fast one on Bubba. One night, Lieutenant Frank Curatola from Battalion Eight was on patrol when he heard a job go down.

Frank was a short, pudgy, big-nosed Italian lad. It was easy to see how he got the nickname Pork Chop, although he could double as the Penguin in a Batman movie. The guy was extremely talented. When he spoke, you could tell he was a fun-loving Italian.

On this night, he decided to "buff" an "unconscious" job. The man deserved credit. He threw on the lights and siren, racing to the call. At the same time, paramedics Joe Hodak and James Patrick "Bubba" Fallar were assigned the job. The race was on.

Frank pulled up first, jumping out running to the back of his vehicle. An older Chinese gentleman was at the door, screaming. Answering the cry for help, our hero Lieutenant Frank flung open the back door in dramatic Hollywood fashion. He had visions of grandeur as he, Lieutenant Frank "Three Tu Da Head" Curatola, would beat the medics and save the patient. With the doors open, it hit him. He, an EMS super supervisor of men and women, had not checked out his vehicle. There was no equipment!

The elderly gentleman was howling and motioning for our hero. Frank wiped his brow as the oil from his slick hair started to run, mixing with his sweat. Frank, never shying away from making command decisions, grabbed for his radio. It went flying out of his slippery hands, landing on the ground.

The old man was motioning in a frenzied manner, babbling for Frank to hurry! Frank found the radio under the rear axle of his vehicle. He picked it up and ran. With radio in hand, a frazzled Lieutenant Frank Curatola climbed the stairs. Placing the radio to his lips, he gasped his distress signal, "Put a rush on da medics!"

This woke up Bubba who was sleeping in the back of the bus.

As they pulled double eight, Joey jumped from the vehicle. Then he helped Bubba who had gotten tangled in his blanket, sheet and straps. Next, they both grabbed the equipment, running into the building. Once in the apartment, they were totally dumbfounded. The "unconscious"—the "Put a rush on da medic!" job—was a leaking, broken water pipe. Bubba summed it all up as he looked at the disheveled lieutenant.

"Hey stupid! You called paramedics for this?"

On July 9, 2000, in Manhattan, a man attacked as Tiffany Goldberg was walking down a street in Manhattan. It was a beautiful day; the energy of the people was accelerating for this young lady. Suddenly, the carefree day was shattered when a man stepped up and smashed the unsuspecting young lady in the head with a large concrete block. The impact was so forceful it not only tore open the skull but sent the victim crashing to the ground. Lying in a pool of blood, totally disoriented, Tiffany looked up to see a man raise the remaining chunk of concrete above his head readying it for the kill. Terrified, unable to scream, she raised her hand. Suddenly, an off-duty fire department lieutenant, Jimmy Hurley, seeing what happened, screamed at the perpetrator and came to her assistance.

Hurley stayed with her, holding her trembling hand, until help arrived, which happened to be coming up the block at that very moment.

Paramedics Tom Reynolds and Arturo Gonzales were cruising their area. They turned onto East Twenty-ninth Street, where the assault had taken place, and pulled up to the scene. Arty went for the immobilization equipment as Tom went to the patient and held stabilization on her profusely bleeding head. The crew treated, packaged and transported her to Bellevue Hospital where she recovered.

End of story. Correct? Wrong. Back at the station, Arty received a phone call from the fire department public relations. The commissioner wanted Arty to make a statement for the press.

It is not uncommon for EMTs or medics to be questioned by the press, although EMS Administration had continually attempted to place a gag order on us going back to the days of Chief Robert Becker. It was fought on our Constitutional rights being violated and won years ago by paramedic Richard McAllen.

Today it's the ego-driven, high-testosterone, no-shame FDNY who still tried to use the "gag" concept, unless of course it brought positive publicity to the FDNY. That, folks, is FDNY, as in firefighters, not EMS.

Thus, the commissioner wanted paramedic Arty Gonzales to state that the fire lieutenant "saved Tiffany Goldberg's life." Arty refused. He said he didn't feel comfortable making such a statement because it wasn't true. At this point, the voice on the other end of the phone got agitated and attempted to order Arty to make the statement. To his credit, Arty still refused.

When EMS people do not cooperate, the FD go to weaker links in the chain. Consequently, Civilian Captain Mark Stone was contacted. In the office, Captain Stone asked what had happened. In front of other crew members, Arty explained, "Upon arriving at the location, the fireman had totally lost it. We had to have him removed by the responding police sector car because he was interfering with patient care. Now the commissioner wants me to say he saved her life."

Evidently not having taken his medication, the good captain got on a conference call and yelled at the commissioner, with his aide and anyone else within earshot, listening. As he reiterated Arty's account, he said, "And what about my paramedics? They, not him, saved her life!"

During a later discussion, Captain Stone confided in me, "As I was yelling, I got a very warm feeling. I stopped and looked up and saw Arty and Tommy standing there, smiling. I put the call on hold. Please, tell me."

Arty looked at him and, over the thunderous roar of laughter, said, "I thought you knew we were kidding."

Captain Mark "I want to be a chief" Stone hit his head against the desk. Between sobs he muttered, "There goes my career. I'll never be chief!"

In reality, the fireman was taken by police car around the neighborhood, looking for the perp. FDNY paramedic Arturo Gonzales made the following statement, "If he was not there, she would have had more blood loss. It was a deep wound." The reality was he didn't do anything medically he was trained to do. But in this instance his actions of yelling and responding saved Tiffany from what might have been her last day on earth.

Headlines on the front page of the Daily News, July 11, 2000, said, "Bash victim's plea: Fireman Jimmy, Don't leave me." The next two pages were about "Hero saves life." For several days, the city was abused and nauseated to death with this over pious reliving of the story. 'Fireman Jimmy' was seen on TV, receiving an award from the mayor, which turned all our stomachs. 'Fireman Jimmy' gave a FDNY sweatshirt to Miss Goldberg. We were all happy for her, but puked when we saw how the world's greatest public relations department, second only to Hollywood, put the spin on for sensation seeking reporters, yet not one damn word about Arty or Tom who medically made the difference. Yeah in today's "free" press the truth dies first which feeds right into the FDNY universe. Gee and you wonder why I watch BBC on channel 13.

Upon hearing the following story, I called the Coney Island garage and left my number. About a day later I received a phone call and was told the story by one of the crew members. The story demonstrates several dangerous flaws in the chain of command.

First, it demonstrates the cluelessness of FDNY brass to run EMS, and the spinelessness of EMS brass to do the right thing. Finally, because of these actions in this case two EMTs almost lost their lives assisting civilians. Because of this policy, based on FDNY ego so crews couldn't monitor or talk to NYPD, lives would indeed be lost.

It started out like any other night in Coney Island. The two EMTs pulled down by the boardwalk and grabbed a breather, enjoying their coffee. The Atlantic's surf rhythmically crashed against the sandy shore. A golden sun was setting, bringing the dusk. It was easy to see why this area was the fun spot for millions of people a year.

The bus was turned off. Its loud, putrid diesel engine no longer belched cloud-polluting air. The invigorating mist from the ocean, Mother Earth's natural rejuvenator, cooled the crew. Whether at Battery Park at the southern end of Manhattan, where Stress Free hung out, or here by the boardwalk in Coney Island, Mother Earth never failed to work her magic on the overworked crews.

On the horizon, the last golden rays intermingled with the dark ocean and the first star of the evening appeared. What a glorious sight. On the other side of the horizon was Great Grandmother Moon, a gigantic full moon, white and gray, making her triumphant entrance.

As the Creator gave the best of life for all to enjoy, they watched, spellbound by the beauty. Suddenly one EMT heard a muffled sound, almost like a cry, followed by laughing. He didn't pay too much attention, figuring it was just kids having fun on the beach. The radio was silent. Since the all-knowing fire department had decided to keep the mixer off, no one could hear each other. The union had brought their safety concerns to the fire commissioner, but the issue fell on deaf ears. Patients in Queens had died because of the mixer-off decision, but the ego-driven Fire Communications Commissioner, Gregory, and his cowering EMS counterpart, David L. Diggs, Chief of Emergency Medical Dispatch, were unmoved.

The commissioner claimed the mixer-off decision was because of the anti-fire statements the crews made, but this was not the case. They re-introduced radio identifiers into the units and no EMS unit was ever charged for anti-fire comments. Once again, one wondered about the validity of anything coming from the fire department.

The union had successfully warded off fire's attempt to take the crystals out of our radios, so we could still monitor and contact the police as needed. Radio contact saved the lives of those who work the streets.

The sound of the seagulls brought the EMT's mind back to the present. Then he heard it again, ever so softly: a muffled sound, a lot of yelling and laughing. Something bothered him. He told his partner, he had a "feeling," a "bad feeling," about the laughing. They decided to follow their instincts, honed on the streets of New York. They got out of the unit to investigate. As they walked, they zipped up their unauthorized, dark blue windbreakers.

The breeze off the ocean was cool on this Indian summer night. The sun was below the horizon, but the moon in all its glory lit the way.

As they moved along the boardwalk, one EMT thought how the Creator had the moon and stars watch over us after the sun went down. He figured it was just the Creator's way of teaching us that no matter how we perceived the Creator, IT always watched over us and would always send someone in the hour of need. We were never alone. The Creator was always with us.

As the crew got closer to the laughing, they heard a girl's muffled cry and scream. Turning down their radios, they cautiously proceeded. The crashing surf drowned out their pounding hearts and cautious steps on the wooden boardwalk. Finally, they spotted the commotion.

A young, white female was stripped naked with her feet being held in the air. A group of fifteen young blacks were taking their turns raping and abusing her. Attempting to squirm free, her legs were held securely by two of the larger males. The crew watched as another male took his turn, dropping his pants and penetrating the helpless girl. Others, waiting their turn, continued to plummet the boyfriend, who was a bloody mass of flesh. He was a defeated spectator. Only able to curse and watch as the pack savagely devoured its catch.

191

The two, Russian Jews, had been enjoying a walk along the boardwalk when the pack approached. As the rape and assault continued, the rabid pack did not notice the two EMTs stealthily approaching. From their safe vantage point behind the wooden benches, the EMTs looked at each other, then the victims. They watched as the attacks became more vicious. The pack was now literally playing with their trapped and wounded victims.

The crew knew if they did not act fast, the victims would be killed. But they were outnumbered and, if discovered, they too could be killed. They had to act and act now. The pounding waves crashed with an increasing sense of urgency.

The words of the great master of warfare, Sun Tzu, thundered in the EMT's head, "Attack should be swift. When an army takes its objective like a hawk striking its prey, and battles like a river broken through a dam, its opponents will scatter before the army tires."

Employing the element of surprise, this army of two, these Street Saints of Compassion, carried their attack forward. They screamed into their radios and at the wild, frenzied pack. Members of the pack yelled "cops" and fled in panic.

The crew members continued the assault, yelling for assistance into their portable radios. But their radios were dead. Silence from the EMS dispatchers.

The crews were smart enough to realize that the element of surprise would soon wear off. The blacks saw two white guys running at them and figured they were cops. But that would not last long. They needed help fast. One EMT switched his radio to the PD frequency and called a 10-13. Some of the young men who ran toward the local projects started to slow. In a few heartbeats, the angry pack started toward the two lone heroes. The two EMTs stood side by side, between the victims and the insane pack. They made their stand.

Suddenly, the streets reverberated with the electrifying sound of sirens as New York's Finest moved in.

It wasn't long before the area was awash with the red and white lights of the police cars and EMS units.

One EMS unit had been sitting only one block away. Because the mixer was turned off, crews could not hear each other. The crew decided to respond on their own when they saw the police pass by.

This story is dedicated to EMTs David Campbell and Ed Lamboy, who were the Army of Two. God does indeed send ordinarily remarkable people to watch over us, so we are never alone.

To establish moral obligation, one needs to have courage. As we have seen, this was greatly lacking in EMS chiefs. At a May meeting of the Health Subcommittee of Community Board Thirteen in Brooklyn, John J. Clair, Assistant Commissioner for Emergency Medicine, sat with Chief McCracken and said that less education is better for EMS crews. This came from a man who failed a medical station at his own EMS refresher. But here's a news flash. In the July 12, 2007 New York Post there was an article that as FDNY assistant commissioner for medical affairs he accepted paid trips, dinners and tickets to "Mamma Mia" from ScanHealth who is doing the billing. Seems his salary wasn't good enough at $109,000. "My acceptance of the gifts was inappropriate," Clair acknowledged. Gee you think? But the more interesting question is where is he working today?

McCracken, for his part, employed three-dollar words like "redynamically" and "redeployment" to lay a smoke screen. He did not want people to discover he was lying through his ass in regard to replacing 33W (paramedic FD unit) with a MetroCare unit, 33U.

In the end, after a powwow with Claire, he admitted he had replaced a unit of city workers with a Giuliani-supported ambulance. Another word—EMS Chief McCracken not only would sacrifice his own people to appease FDNY, but was a liar.

As the Peanut Gallery gave away the house, we paupers went on. FDNY was learning the hard way they got a handful with "those EMS people."

Sometimes us EMS people would have a little fun at the fire department's expense. I know the following individual very well since in the "old days" we enjoyed McDonnell's together on more than one occasion.

A certain EMS captain was decked out in his new fire department uniform, alone on patrol in the borough. He observed a fire engine parked in front of a call. The chauffeur stood beside the truck, as the EMS captain approached, "What are you just standing around for?" he asked the startled fireman.

"Sir, the crew is upstairs with a cardiac call, helping *those EMS people*," he proudly said.

"Do you want to go to BITS along with your whole engine company?" demanded the captain, confusing the fireman.

"No sir."

"Then read regulation 1-2105 that was just put out by the commissioner.

It says, 'The chauffeur, that's you, is to open all fire hydrants at the scene of the call. This will increase productivity, by checking the hydrants at full pressure while the engine is assisting *those EMS people*.'"

No one can ever say these firemen aren't smart, I mean able to follow orders...blindly.

As the captain drove away and looked in his rear view mirror, a smile crossed his face. Two fire hydrants blasted away, flooding the street as the chauffeur looked for a third.

Within a day, the fire gods knew they were had. They ordered a change in uniforms so their firemen could tell the difference between a fire officer and *those EMS people*.

This broke the hearts of the civilian EMS chiefs, who thought they were like the big boys in the department.

To further show their paranoia, on January 5, 1998, they changed EMS' designation from Bureau of EMS to

EMS Command, command being of lesser prestige. EMS was reduced from bureau, a higher rank, to command, a lower rank. By the way, our hero EMS captain was never caught.

Still, the Fidney Paupers continued in their quest to provide the best care possible to our public. Below is another story about paramedic Tom Reynolds that shows the lengths some of our paramedics and EMTs go.

One day, Tom had an elderly lady who refused to go to the hospital for reasons unknown. Both Tom and his partner felt the patient's condition warranted the trip. Nothing either crew member said made a difference. Finally, Tom called his mom.

His partner stood in shock as Tom explained to Mom what was going on and the patient's refusal to go to the hospital. Tom handed the phone to the woman, advising her, "My mom wants to talk to you." After several minutes, she gave the phone back. Tom's mom convinced the elderly woman to go to the hospital. We now call her Telemetry Mom.

But now let's see an example of why it's important to have the mixer on so units can hear each other in regard to patient care.

I was working a Basic unit years ago in Spanish Harlem when the dispatcher blared, "Fourteen Boy, you have a 'pedestrian struck.'" Certain things are guaranteed on this job. The worst job will always be at the end of the tour, when you are about to go home. And the "difficult breather" will always be three hundred pounds, in an apartment on the top floor, at the end of the hall, with the elevator out of service. The job was at One Hundred Sixth Street. My partner and I responded.

As we pulled up to the address, people were screaming. I could see the legs of a four-year-old child pinned under a car. A lone blood-soaked sneaker lay away from the unmoving child. As my partner jumped out, I attempted to call for medics.

"Emergency! Emergency! Fourteen Boy Emergency!" Everyone cleared the air. "Location, One Hundred Sixth Street, cross, Second to Third. I have an unresponsive child pinned and need medics. Copy Central?"

By announcing an emergency, I knew the crews would listen. By giving the location and disposition of a child, I knew units would come to help without the dispatcher assigning them. The days of the quality of dispatcher were long over.

Tommy Young was dispatching and I got no response. Finally, he came on. "Listen, dick. Relax. I have jobs to hand out and then I'll get to you medics!"

Did I hear what I thought I heard? This was a statement I did not need to hear.

"Want to repeat that again, hero?" I asked.

"Yeah, dick. You heard me." Now this is too much. But the dispatchers have always been the sacred cows of EMS, and I do mean cows.

"Would you like to discuss this after the job?" I countered.

"Come on down, dick." was his response.

Before he could assign any units, a medic as well as several Basic units, had "buffed" the job, claiming to be "flagged" at the scene. Buffing is not waiting to be called. Flagged is claiming you stumbled upon the job. Working the streets, we learned not to depend on dispatchers when the chips are down, but on ourselves.

We needed all the units to assist in both utilizing the crowd and literally lifting the vehicle so as to release the child. It never ceased to amaze me that people, even in emotionally chaotic, life-and-death situations involving a child always could be put to good use once organized. The folks of Spanish Harlem were no different, following our directions as the Dance of Life started.

As I assisted the medics, everyone said the same thing, "I can't believe he said that over the air."

"You heard him invite me out there, right?"

"Yeah, we sure did."

Thanks to all concerned, the child survived, though permanent brain damage would make his life tough. It was the end of my tour as I walked outside the hospital, and Tommy Young was still on the radio.

"Fourteen Boy Central," I said into the radio.

"Fourteen Boy," he came back.

"ETA to your location twenty minutes. I'm taking you up on your offer."

He responded, "I'll be waiting, dick."

This was just going to be too easy and deeply enjoyable, I thought, pulling into Metropolitan Hospital, our garage. My final act was, "Fourteen Boy, ETA fifteen minutes." Tommy Young was off the radio. The new dispatcher responded, "I will gladly give him the message." Unknown to me at the time, the dispatchers were taking bets on how many bones I'd break with one shot.

Meanwhile, Mr. EMT, Tom Young, sat safely cowering next to the useless tour commander in a separate office. When you are dealing with a bunch of wannabe paramilitary types, it really takes the challenge out of it.

I pulled up to the front of Puzzle Palace, Location One in Maspeth, Queens. The Hop Cops, hospital cops, were standing at the entrance.

They were waiting for me. The only problem was they did not know what I looked like.

The idiot floor lieutenants and tour commander told them that I would be pulling up in my ambulance. You know what they say about assumptions.

So, pulling up in my little red Honda, I waved and the hop cops waved back. Then I pulled around to the back. Those frontal assaults are okay for the United States Marines, but being an army paratrooper I would rather use my brain and go the way of least resistance. So after parking around back, I walked in through the bay area, saying hello to all. I walked down a long corridor and past a room filled with dispatchers and a lieutenant named Ike. I had met him once at Bellevue. Being himself, he got off on the wrong foot with me.

Thus we were already acquainted. Everyone turned as I walked by.

"Hi," I said with a smile.

"Hi," came the reply. About six steps past the door, I heard them scream in unison, "Schrang!"

Couldn't put much past these geniuses! The office rapidly emptied and dear Lieutenant Ike requested my audience.

"Okay," I said, "but then I'll talk to Mr. Young."

Once inside, Ike started running off at the mouth without his brain in gear and still in his ass, just like the first time I met him. I guess consistency counts for something.

"I'm going to get you fired!"

"Never make promises you can't keep."

Looking at the duty captain, then back to me, he said, "You drove out here in an ambulance you stole from Metropolitan Hospital and went into two different boroughs with it."

Okay, so now the genius was giving a mapping class. Howdy Doody here was confirming my belief that he wasn't related to General 'Ike' Eisenhower because at least the later knew how to read a map.

"No, I drove out here in my little red Honda," I said calmly, which cranked him.

Flustered, both looked at each other before Ike retorted, "You are here on HHC (Health and Hospital Corporation) property illegally!" Gee, this guy was turning so red I bet if the lights went out I'd still see him, I thought.

"No, your dispatcher, Mr. Young, invited me out over the radio."

I could no longer hide my smile. Hell, if this was a battle of brains they were clearly demonstrating they were totally unarmed!

Okay, this guy and his wannabes were having a bad day. Thus they decided to push the issue upstairs.

In a less than professional manner he proclaimed, "You stay here. I'm calling the chief!"

Gee, doesn't that sound like, "You wait here! I'm calling your father!"?

From a phone in an adjacent office he called Chief Gustav Pappas, who was in charge of communications.

"Chief Pappas is on the phone," proclaimed the good lieutenant, sounding like a two-year-old.

"Pick it up!"

After that last statement, I guess he found some Miracle Grow and grew a pair.

"Hello," I said in a weary voice, the fun of dealing with Twiddle Dee and Twiddle Dumber was really old and I still hadn't met Mr. Young yet.

"Jim, what are you up to?" Chief Pappas asked, trying to hide a chuckle.

"Oh, I'm here to kill one of your dispatchers for cursing me out on the air."

Gus now openly chuckled.

"Listen, do me a favor."

"Sure."

"Write up what happened and send it to me. I'll take care of him, okay?"

"Sure, no problem, chief."

"Please put Lieutenant Ike on. Thanks."

Ike and his little cohort were listening in. I clicked the receiver down, then up, and listened.

These clowns were real losers.

"Do you want us to have him arrested?" the good lieutenant asked.

Gus answered, "No way. You'd really have a problem then."

"Well, can I suspend him from duty?"

Gus had about as much as I had.

"Look! I'm going home. Leave Schrang alone. He will forward me the paperwork."

Click. I smiled, put the phone on the receiver, and started to walk out.

"Where do you think you're going?" Lieutenant Ike asked.

"I'm going to work. So have a nice day," Pushing past him and out the door. I did as requested by Chief Pappas. What Twiddle Dee and Twiddle Dumber did not realize was that Gus Pappas was my instructor in an EMT course at Saint Vincent's Hospital many years ago. Even further back, we became part of a blood brotherhood—the brotherhood of combat Vietnam veterans. This bond had always served us well.

Once in a refresher course, Gus cracked a joke about army paratroopers. I excused myself and left the class. Upon returning, as the instructor was speaking, I nailed Gus with an extra large cup of water and passed a remark about his naval career with the marines. Next to Big Bird, Chief Maniscalco, Gus was another renegade the establishment burned in more than one way.

After forwarding the report to Gus, I contacted the FCC in lower Manhattan realizing Gus would keep his word, but not the EMS god. I dealt a preemptive strike. Later, I was informed that EMS communications did a "President Nixon" on the tape. The tape of our conversation was "lost." However, they did pay a hefty fine and Mr. Young was out of communications.

Several months later, as I pulled into Bellevue I saw an EMT and asked who he was.

"Oh that's Tommy Young," my partner said with a snicker. I jumped out of the vehicle and approached.

"Young!" I yelled. He was drinking Coke through a straw.

"Yeah. Who wants to know?" sounding really tough, until I said the key word.

"Schrang!" He almost choked on the drink.

"Want to finish our business now, asshole?" I queried.

"Uh, I'm sorry," he meekly said, putting out his hand for me to shake.

"Don't ever say anything over a radio you don't have the balls to back up in person." I warned, leaving his hand in midair.

200

A year or two later we were in the same paramedic class at the academy. Tommy was a potbellied lieutenant at Bellevue. One night a dispatcher was talking to him on the radio. I guess she had the hots for the butterball.

"Gee, I was just told you used to be a dispatcher here," she coyly stated.

"Yeah, I couldn't wait to get out of there."

With this I broke in from Stress Free, my paramedic unit, "Then you should have asked me earlier, Tommy," I said. He went hysterically crazy with laughter.

Lieutenant, wish I could find my brain Ike was still in communications. One night threatening a dispatcher because she said "thank you" to a unit on the radio telling her he would give her a CD if she said it again. Ah, consistency is important.

There are paramedics who walk among us, who go above and beyond to answer the call of humanity. Three NYC EMS paramedics are people of such extraordinary character. They answered the call to go to Bosnia with me. I had been going to Bosnia on humanitarian missions since 1993. In May 1995, Michael Nunnery of Rhode Island and I formed Life Mission and were running trips. Mike did prosthetics and I took care of the EMS side.

Three NYC paramedics, Rachel Barney, Eric Lonergan, and Richard Stein, went on a month-long mission, late summer of 1995. All three paid their own fares. They walked the streets of Sarajevo, coming under heavy fire from Serbian antiaircraft guns.

Back in the States, I forwarded a letter to the Awards Committee via Captain Mark Stone. Chief McCracken acknowledged receiving it and passed it on. The committee did not feel it relevant to acknowledge these three New York City paramedics for their professionalism, unselfishness, humanitarianism, and compassion. Instead, they glorified several medics who went on a paid trip to Russia to bestow thirty thousand dollars of equipment donated by another agency.

I could care less about awards and decorations for myself since Mike and I had the satisfaction of knowing what we accomplished for the people of Bosnia with paramedic heroes like James Dawdy III of Arizona and these three special people from New York City. Still, it hurt that they were totally ignored.

The last I heard Rachel went on to become a Marine chopper pilot, Eric a doctor, and Richie died. I'm honored to have served with them all.

Eight
The Cost
Liars, Thieves, and Victims

"EMS is not for everyone, no matter what your devotion to service. It requires a special person to have the courage to accept the responsibility of life-and-death decisions in emergency circumstances." Mayor Rudy Giuliani, in his eulogy for Christopher Prescott, Holy Child R.C. Church on June 20, 1994.

In the lonely, wee hours of the morning, when you are safely asleep in warm beds, the Street Saints of Compassion are not. They are watching over you.

It was such a morning on June 17, 1994, when on the corner of Eastern Parkway and Utica Avenue in Brooklyn, EMT Christopher Prescott and his partner, EMT Carol Buffer, had their final job together. At about 1:30 a.m. as they worked to save others a drunk brought death and untold pain to the crew members. In a split second, Chris was traumatically crushed and Carol was in critical condition. Our sister, Carol, fought for her life and survived. This was an incident the civilian gods and the city government could not sweep under the rug. The crew's blood baptized the street and reminded us that the Street Saints of Compassion have sacred and dangerous jobs.

EMT Christopher Prescott was the first EMS professional to die in the line of duty by a drunk driver.

On November 1, 1989, EMT Tracy Allen Lee became the first EMS professional to die of AIDS contracted on the job. She had worked out of Bellevue and I always remember the twinkle in her eye and big, gregarious smile.

On that fateful day Tracy and her partner responded to a job in a SRO hotel on Thirty-fourth Street in Manhattan. The location was known as the AIDS Hotel, since all the guests were HIV positive, compounded with other medical problems such as TB, cardiac, mental, drug, alcohol, asthma, and the like.

When the crew got there, they worked the patient, who was bleeding. Tracy reportedly cut her hand on a nail, as she moved the patient into position. With disregard for her own safety, she continued the Dance of Life, for this stranger.

Later, she realized the patient's blood and body fluid had entered her through her nicked thumb. She reported it to a supervisor, completed an official exposure report and then was gone. EMS administration did a good job at keeping the fact hidden. When asking about her condition all the crews would be told was "she is out on sick leave." Nothing more was told until she reached out to the union, which got word to the crews. I never did see Tracy again.

In May of 1994, it was confirmed she had AIDS. From that point on, the nightmare began for this gentle soul. The city would not budge. Now blind in one eye, Tracy watched the funeral of Princess Diana of England and spoke of the passing of Mother Teresa, whom she had seen in the South Bronx. She referred to both as angels. Within eighteen days, EMT Tracy Allen Lee was dead.

The city would not honor her request for a letter acknowledging she received her death sentence from the job. When Judge Jay Liebowitz ruled in Tracy's favor, the city appealed. Tracy got no resolution.

At Tracy's funeral, the hypocrites still could not give her rest. Mayor Giuliani stood beside the coffin, singing her praises, yet it was his administration that tortured the girl to the end with its appeals. The only reason Mayor Giuliani, the fire gods, and the EMS chiefs were there was because they feared a public relations firestorm.

Tracy left behind a letter; in part it said, "Saving lives is so important and I want each of you to promise to stay safe and be careful. In peace now. Tracy."

We had the best angel in Tracy.

The caring Giuliani administration did not settle with the Lee family until eighteen months *after her death*. This EMS professional was mortally wounded on a job attempting to save a stranger's life, yet she was treated worse than a criminal. Criminals have rights. Tracy filled out the official exposure report as most of us have, but an unsympathetic mayor and fire department engaged in character assassination. Yet, three fire chiefs were "retired on disability," each to draw more than $100,000 annually, tax free, for the rest of their lives.

One complained he had acquired "a hearing impairment" through the years. Guess what? I too have a hearing impairment, as well as many of my brothers and sisters, caused by listening to the sirens. Where are our payoffs?

Below are direct quotes from the Fire God himself, Thomas Von Essen, from the "Commissioner's Message" in Fire Works, May 2000.

"Recently, a (fire) lieutenant, not wearing his bunker pants, was burned seriously on his legs. He lied and said he had them on. Some of the people who work for Chief Ganci and me wanted to give him charges. He certainly deserved charges. We told him to tell the truth and change the reports. He did and now is retired on disability.

In a recent fire, a firefighter went to the fire floor, the second, and seriously injured his lungs. He lied and said he took the stairs when actually he used the elevator. We had a videotape of him using the elevator.

He is retired on disability. No charges of fraud, attempting to deceive, no charges—period."

These two firemen lied; one was an officer. They falsified documents and submitted fraudulent claims, hiding their own stupidity in receiving the injuries. One of the firefighters injured his lungs, and management complained about his elevator use. He did not get damaged lungs by riding an elevator, but by not using the protective gear, in this case the Scott Pack with portable air.

The commissioner advised them to change the reports and all was forgiven. So he compounded the lie.

Tracy Allen Lee never lied, never changed a document or made a fraudulent claim. Nor did she suffer her mortal wound due to stupidity. What did she get? Shit, with phony sympathy from the mayor and Fire God. In the fire world, lying is an accepted trait. What else did the New York City Fire Department promise?

In 1996, FDNY told the city council there would be close to sixty new EMS stations built. To date there are four, Harlem, Astoria, Woodhull and Elmhurst.

In the Commissioner's Message, in Fire Works, March 2000, he said, "Both EMTs and paramedics equally have the opportunity to be promoted to lieutenant (a $20.00-a-week raise over top paramedic), or opt to take the promotion exam to become a firefighter." You know what I thought of this.

In pre-merger days, the EMS command ran 122 ALS (paramedic) tours and 385 BLS (EMT) tours for a total of 507 tours. Post-merger, the EMS command ran 139 ALS tours and 444 BLS tours, a 16 percent increase in total tours. He forgot to mention these tours were the result of mandating crews, to the point where they were *exhausted and quit*.

Look at the environment in which Tracy and the rest of us work. Do you see a double standard, or is it just me?

According to information provided by Local 2507, since the merger of EMS and fire, FDNY Personnel Director, Ms. Sherry Kavaler, had fired hundreds of EMTs and paramedics. Many were due to medical reasons, like the fireman's lung problems, or back problems from lifting patients, as opposed to casserole dishes in a firehouse. For every EMT or paramedic who retired from the service, seven or eight were fired or resigned.

The situation was almost exactly the reverse among the uniformed ranks. The overwhelming majority of firefighters made it through their twenty years to retirement. Ms. Kavaler's numerous termination letters had earned her the sobriquet "The Terminator."

So much for Commissioner Von Essen's statement that the reason for mandating was, "Every day people are going sick with 'exhaustion' after being assigned overtime."

The Terminator fired people for medical problems and the Fire God complained because people were sick and exhausted from mandated overtime.

Sooner or later this will lead to a deficit and the system will crash.

The EMS Academy is located at historic Fort Totten in Bayside, New York. Some thought it to be a sacred Native American burial site. A sensitive paramedic reported "hearing voices" she believed to be Native American. After talking to me, she honored them with sage offerings one night.

Once past the security post, a winding road lazily meandered upward into a tree-lined road. To the right sat a black antiaircraft crew served weapon from a time period not too long ago and a tribute to man's belief in the insanity of separation, domination, hatred, and death. On the grass during the fall season, one would walk between numerous friendly Canadian geese, which flocked to this location for hundreds of years, celebrating life. To the left, just before one enters the shade of the trees just past now-abandoned World War Two ammunition bunkers, was the Little Bay. A long, jagged stone jetty stretched into the bay from which people fished during the summer. Further out, dominating the blue skyline, Throgs Neck Bridge majestically arched across the East River, uniting, providing life's blood to the people of Queens and Bronx boroughs. At the fork, if one continued straight, were the remains of the original fort used against the British during the Revolutionary War, long since chain-fenced off, forgotten and discarded. My journey took me to the right, deeper into the caressing, tree-lined road. Sweet fragrances combined with birds' lyrical singing voices, the resulting vibrations a melody celebrating life. At the top of the hill to the left sat a manicured parade field surrounded on all sides by full, ancient trees, basking in rays of the early morning sun. From here I could see the red brick and gray roof of the EMS Academy. It was where the finest EMTs and paramedics in the world had graduated, but it was also a living tribute of knowledge celebrating life. This was the birthplace of the Dance of Life we EMS people perform each day, serving the public.

Our scores on the New York State Exam, taken every three years, proved it. We led the state and pushed up the average, thanks to the mentors and pioneers we called instructors.

Paramedics like Rudy Havelka, Debbie Monte, David Russell, Toni Lanotte, Carl Tramontana, Manuel Delgado, Tom Carlstrom, Willie Silvestry, and, of course, "Mom" Lori Santo.

These people were not just the best in NYC EMS, but in the world. Their quest for perfection was reflected not only in test scores but, more importantly, in the quality of the paramedics on the streets of New York.

These were the days before the Fire God ruined the academy. During the CFR program, a dictate came down from the mayor's office that "no fireman would fail." This did not sit well with a lot of the instructors, who could not be intimidated. One instructor had failed a complete engine company because they couldn't or wouldn't master the skills. Skills that I might add a junior high school student could pass and that these firefighters were getting paid overtime for. As a disciplinary measure he, the instructor was transferred to 9 Metro Tech (Puzzle Palace) the next morning. Many other instructors transferred or were transferred.

The academy had been the foundation of EMS. By demanding excellence, the instructors forced the EMTs and paramedics to shine on the streets of New York. The instructors were as vital to EMS as blood is to the human body. Silently, the EMS civilian chiefs stood by as the very foundation of EMS, the academy, was torn asunder, gutted. Did you expect less?

During my last refresher course, I reflected on the academy, what it had been and how it deteriorated under EMT Robert McCracken, civilian Chief of EMS Command, and John J. Claire, Assistant Commissioner for Emergency Medicine. In short, they aided and abetted the destruction of the academy.

Lieutenant David Russell worked hard to put together a fantastic physical fitness program and gym. The gym alone would make Arnold Schwarzenegger proud. As Dave worked to get the equipment, he also did his research and put together a program. After all this, the fire department replaced him with a fireman, not on a truck.

I took my last exam in the building they used for the CFR Program down the block from the EMS Academy. As I entered the front door, the atmosphere changed as a gaunt, rum-nosed fireman stoically pointed to a sign directing me to the classroom. That morning I recalled seeing a TV reporter interview two of CFR demonstrating basic first aid for the interview. They unabashedly stated, "We save the person's life, the ambulance comes to transport."

I stopped to observe wall-to-wall, ceiling-to-ceiling citations of "saves" by FD doing medical jobs. Bold letters blared, "Engine so-and-so saved," then, a summary of the job. At the bottom of the page, in very small print,

"Ambulance so-and-so on scene," then the time was shown. I glanced back at the fireman, and chuckled, thinking the wall is worth no more than the egotistical phony propaganda pinned to it. I guess next, each engine will have four cameramen and one fireman...or has that already come to be?

During the refresher, I learned that FD was considering hiring a dean and turning the facility into the "College of Fire and Life."

They were looking at an individual from Harvard. The concept was fantastic. This could have an extremely positive effect on the fire department's ability to provide the world's best integrated model of fire suppression and EMS in the world. The pluses would emanate from a highly educated force, pushing the envelope of excellence in both the fire and pre-hospital medical fields. Technology advancements would provide cutting-edge, cost-effective means of saving lives. The people of New York stood to gain much. This integrated force could also bring in revenues by sending crews outside CONUS (continental United States) to teach, as well as provide formal training at Fort Totten.

The reality was, to have such a world-renowned Mecca, it had to exemplify true integration, and I'm not only talking about those who were not Irish, or Italian. Nature, from the trees, to the snow geese, to the spirits of Native Americans who still roamed the grounds, demonstrated that creativity is wrought from the unity of diversity, not separation which man projects. Could FDNY Administration learn so all prosper? Little by little, the pace accelerated as the top brass got rid of, or forced out, the best EMS instructors in the world demonstrating that they didn't have a clue as to the treasure they were destroying.

Still, the question begged an answer, why would they require a guy carrying a hose, putting wet stuff on the red stuff, to have a degree, unless it was to keep out minorities? It couldn't be that since their callous, unabashed track record against EMS had demonstrated their anti-minority stance repeatedly. Or did it go even deeper than this? The commissioner had balked at allowing paramedics advance their education by becoming physician assistants or even registered nurses. He claimed we should take the promotional exam to become firefighters.

Considering our education, playing with a hose is not a step up, but down. Yet when EMS people did apply for the promotional exam, that's an in-house exam a large percentage blatantly denied. Interestingly enough we heard rumors that both the fire commissioners son as well as chief

McCraken's sons didn't have a problem being appointed. Why then the push for educating the Bravest if you were not accepting the more highly educated department members? Why someone from Harvard?

Think about it. They destroyed the educated half of the fire department, EMS, whose members are the life's blood to over a million people a year. The commissioner blocked every effort of the union to gain uniform status for us or allow us to increase our educational base of knowledge. The uneducated brothers fighting decreasing numbers of fires and spending more and more time idly were now going to have a school to gain a Ph.D. in Fire Science. It sure didn't make sense to me, until I used a time-proven suggestion that sank Al Capone and was later told by Deep Throat to two reporters during the Nixon Water Tape scandal *"Follow the money."* Yes gentle reader investigator reporters did once exist in the now void canned thoughtless commercialized dimwitted news world.

A new facility called FDNY Fire Zone, located at 34 West Fifty-first Street between Fifth and Sixth Avenues, opened in October 2000. The February 1, 2001 edition of the Civilian Bulletin, Bureau of Personnel Resources, Volume XI, Issue No. 3, published by the fire department, ran an interesting article. It stated, "There is an official FDNY store offering specially designed FDNY T-shirts, baseball caps, jackets, and more. These are officially licensed FDNY products, and sold exclusively at the Fire Zone. All proceeds go into the Fire Safety Education Fund to support operation of Fire Zone and FDNY Fire Safety programs."

Yet The Fire Zone has not one thing about EMS. This would be a great place to teach the public about health emergencies and educate the public about vital signs, EKGs, and the like. But, of course, the focus would then be on public welfare and knowledge base, not FDNY ego.

Firefighters work at the Fire Zone. Once again, how many are on the trucks? We see firefighters, running gyms, and doing light duty for ten years. Some work on the tire truck. Now we have them running a profit making, ego-driven facility. They hand out belt buckles and are in charge of the computer section.

Deputy Commissioner Frank Gribbon, a spokesman for the Fire Department, said the billing unit was beefed up from five (Remember there are five men on a truck), to fifty people. It seemed that FDNY "lost" close to $40 million! First, doesn't their charter with the City say something about *not charging for services*? Well, it does, but the Giuliani Administration realized that EMS and DOT were the only two money-making, not losing, agencies in city government. Thus FDNY would bill for EMS, reaping the profits, if they could count that high. Because this blunder brought an investigative eye on FDNY billing practices, we, EMS crews, were ordered to report to the academy, lectured and threatened to fill out our ACRs with "billing insurance information." Not once was patient care mentioned, rather billing information, and how we would "lose days" if we failed to comply. FDNY didn't staff their billing department correctly, didn't give EMS appropriate funding from their newly inflated budget, and we the crews get lectured, then threatened.

What is their next excuse? Talking about budgets, here is an example, suppose the fire suppression side responded to three hundred thousand calls and EMS did 1.3 million calls, an average of over 3,000 calls in a twenty-four-hour period. We have actually gone over four thousand already. By combining the two, FDNY now will ask for a budget increase for close to two million calls a year. Since they are the governing agency, they now allocate the money to EMS, and, trust me, we have come up short.

Also, I really have to hand it to you by opening up those multi-million-dollar deals with the big apartment stores to sell the official FDNY hats and T-shirts. Seems you didn't lose track here.

Once again I have a problem. It seems I'm a problem-type guy. Not that you made the deal. No, I have a problem with you going after honest, hardworking immigrants selling the bootlegged brand.

Also, how many damn commissioners and assistant commissioners to the commissioners do you need to put *wet stuff on the red stuff?* The only thing I see being beefed up is the upper crust of the FDNY and *unaccountability of money. Where is this money going?*

EMT Denise Chapman responded to a job in the Bronx. She found an intoxicated male, reeking of feces, urine, and covered with bugs. Without hesitation, she and her partner did their jobs. As the patient was being moved from their stretcher to one at Lincoln Hospital, bugs went flying in all directions. The staff at the Lincoln Hospital confirmed the patient had tuberculosis. The next morning, she was still pulling ticks from her skin. "I had ticks and lice all over me," she stated to me in an interview.

Denise completed the official exposure report. For six months, the fire department doctors at BHS sent her home sick with headaches and vomiting. Not once did they do any tests, until an outside physician performed a skin test for tuberculosis. Only then did the medical geniuses decide to take x-rays and do sputum tests. Only after she was referred to a psychiatrist for evaluation did she finally receive a blood test, confirming she had contracted Lyme disease. You would think BHS would start to move on her case, right? Wrong.

March 13, 1997. Denise filed for worker's compensation and LODI. LODI was denied and the city law department controverted the case. Denise filed a complaint against the fire department through the New York State Department of Labor's Public Employee Safety and Health Bureau (PESH). The result was that the Bravest were cited by PESH for safety and health violations. Even with the official exposure report and documentation of Lyme disease-carrying ticks in Bronx's Van Cortland Park and blood tests, Denise was denied worker's compensation benefits.

July 1997. Local 2507 President Kevin Lightsey requested Fire Commissioner Thomas Von Essen to grant LODI to Denise. He never responded.

213

The following year, Executive Board Member Richard McAllen of the local sent a follow-up letter. The only thing returned from the commissioner of the Bravest was silence. The same death knell that killed EMT Tracy Allen Lee.

March 18, 1998. Denise received a letter from fire department Personnel Director Sherry Ann Kavaler, "The Terminator," firing her.

August 1999. The New York State Department of Labor informed Local 2507 that they sustained a complaint and agreed the fire department had retaliated against Denise after she filed a health and safety complaint two years prior. According to Inspector Raynard Caines, PESH was in the process of forwarding the case to the New York State Attorney General.

November 2000, I asked Denise's permission to use this information. She graciously gave it. After losing her apartment, car, savings, but most of all, her health, she was concerned that this should not happen to another member of NYC EMS.

This young, talented Street Saint of Compassion now lived in her mother's house. She had a lifeport in her chest and IV bags attached. She was sensitive to light, had constant headaches, dizziness, muscle weakness, and joint pain. Unable to work, she was dependent on public assistance. All of this due to the Lyme disease she contracted on the job, a disease that, if identified and treated aggressively with antibiotics, could have been neutralized. The Fire God must feel real proud.

In the latest update from Denise, I learned her doctor's office caught fire, burning mainly her records. She spoke to Fire Marshall Joseph Pascarello, who seemed extremely interested in the case, until she explained her situation with the fire department. Suddenly, he closed the case, like a red-hot door. Even her doctor was growing less interested in the case since she heard rumors he was being "pressured" before the fire nearly destroyed his practice.

Coincidence? How come all FDNY records for her case were missing when PESH investigated? After the records disappeared, Ellis Oliver, a 2507 Union Representative who confirmed to Denise the disappearance of the station log and Infectious Exposure books, stopped calling her. Help from Local 2507 died.

When PESH finally reopened the investigation, all the records were gone. Even her TB exposure record was lost, and FD Dr. Prizant claimed amnesia. Unfortunately for him, Denise still had the bottle of medicine he had prescribed for her.

Denise wrote to me, "I know Frank Mineo of FDNY was involved with this in the beginning. After he left, who knows? And Thomas Galvin and his assistant had something to do with this. Galvin also is no longer there. Bello, supervisor from PESH, is gone. Coincidence? I don't think so. I know this was no accident. I am scared."

Wouldn't FDNY and their insurance company lose a lot of money paying long-range care to treat people like Denise? After all, the FDNY screwed up by not getting her the appropriate care in the beginning. *Again we are talking about money,* a common haunting question when dealing with FDNY. Please recall, current post 9-11 problems mentioned earlier in the book. Again, it's about the money and second class citizenship.

Denise did not lie, falsify documents, or get injured because of stupidity. The fire commissioner claims to be a man who can make tough decisions. Well here is a no-brainer, even for him. He awarded pensions to *his brothers* despite lies, falsification of documentation, and stupidity. Denise did her job, yet he refused to even entertain her case. Seems like a double standard to me.

On April 7, 1997, staff writer Joe Calderone wrote an article in the Daily News entitled; "Bravest Brass Go for the Gold." It stated that five fire department chiefs were about to be demoted so they decided to retire.

Instead of just retiring, these five heroes decided to put in for disability pensions.

"Each is contending that line of duty injuries (LODI) make them unable to continue their jobs." They worked with no problems, until they were to be demoted. Then they claimed their injuries rendered them unable to continue their jobs. How do we spell fraud?

One of the heroes, fifty-eight-year-old Division Commander Salvatore Sansone, who applied for a disability pension of $115,402 a year, tax free, stated to the reporter, "You are foolish if you don't {apply} because those {pension} laws are in place."

The article went on to report that more than "Ten chiefs have cashed out in recent years, each with tax-free disability pensions in excess of $100,000, including the department's former Chief Medical Officer, Dr. Cyril Jones."

The fire department pension "covers for cancer, heart, and lung problems—even if there is no direct evidence linking the injury to the job." Evidence? But that's only for firefighters.

This should make Denise feel better, if her vision is still good enough to read it. According to a union official, firefighters routinely prepare for retirement by filing for disability pensions, even if their injuries occurred long ago and far from a fire. Jon Sorensen of the Daily News reported this information. Each of the above heroes was in a high-level post, so the question came up as to when they received their injuries. Sansone applied because of hearing loss in his right ear, plus neck and heart ailments.

Another hero, Division Commander James Corcoran, whose annual pension would be $114,715, said doctors at BHS picked up possible lung disease. This is the same BHS that did not do a damn thing for Denise, but "lose" her records.

Corcoran went on to state, "If you have a problem with your lungs, you are entitled to be considered. It's not as if they are handing you something for nothing. Thirty-four years in the fire department is a lot of smoke." Yeah, he can sure blow smoke up some civilian, white-collar, or child's ass, but not ours.

How many pictures are there of the Bravest working at a fire with their Scott Packs, oxygen bottles, off? Why does the city allow a disability if they aren't using the equipment? Oh, I forgot, silly me. You need your face clear for the photos.

According to EMS regulations, EMTs and paramedics are to be two floors below an active fire. Thus if this hero is claiming a disability that the quacks at BHS just discovered, I'm one up on him. At my last medical, I learned I had hearing and lung loss. Where is my pension? We are not issued Scott Packs. If we do not go to a floor as commanded, we are found guilty of insubordination and refusing a lawful order.

Realizing the fraud, two people—and only two people with integrity— tried to correct this. Former State Senator Michael Holblock, a Republican from Albany, and Assemblywoman Audrey Hochberg, a Democrat from Scarsdale, attempted to make a difference. According to an article dated April 8, 1997, both of their bills succumbed to the might of the well-greased firefighters' lobby. Governor Pataki said he is seeking new limits, but his bill exempts New York City firefighters.

I do not wish to deny the very best to any firefighter who is injured or killed in the line of duty. But I do expect people like Denise and others to be taken care of. Firemen do not face death each day. The fact is, the number of fires is down. Most firemen today have not been exposed to fires like those in Brooklyn in the early eighties or the burning of the Bronx in the seventies, but more about this later when you read what happened post 9-11.

One article stated that a firefighter was awarded a tax-free disability pension because he hurt his back raising a flag. Another got a disability pension because he was injured carrying a casserole in a firehouse kitchen. Bravest, I think not. Another of the brothers, on disability, ran a marathon in the Empire State Building.

With regard to Division Commander Salvatore Sansone's egotistical statement, "You are foolish if you don't apply," I say that when the Street Saints of Compassion have an unconscious patient, 99.9 percent of us know not to take his wallet or jewelry. The trust is there, built on reputation. We can't say the same for the New York City Fire Department whose reputation is built on the claims of their fraudulent disability pensions. It would appear to me that money speaks louder to them than integrity. Oh, and just a side note, not one face of color were among these heroes who bailed out.

Everyday, EMS crews are threatened with death. We deal with the sick, the emotionally disturbed, gunshot victims, SIDS babies, overdoses, AIDS patients, and the like. I demand better for my people.

Paramedic James Patrick "Bubba" Fallar was attending his refresher course on March 1, 1999. Unlike other surrounding states, which are set up in a more professional framework for EMTs and paramedics with competent Continuing Medical Education (CME), in backward New York City we have to take a state test every three years. If we fail, we get another shot, but if we fail again, then we are out of a job. Paramedics, unlike EMTs, get the distinct pleasure of taking yet another exam, the Regional Emergency Medical Advisory Committee (REMAC), so we can work in the city. But there is no stress on the job, right?

Thanks to the fire department and no thanks to the doctors hiding in the Office of Medical Affairs, we have less time off the streets for refresher courses. Most EMTs and paramedics looked forward to this time, not only to fine-tune their skills and learn something new, but it also served as a badly needed psychological break from the streets. Remember, two EMS members from the Federal Building attack committed suicide because of the stress. To reiterate, we respond to over three thousand calls in twenty-four hours. Thus a refresher serves a vital mental health service not provided for.

Studies in Canada, England, and the States show at least 20 percent of crew members suffer from Post Traumatic Stress Syndrome. A recent study by the Los Angeles Fire Department, reported by Kurt Streeter, a Los Angeles Times staff writer, had some interesting data. The study focused on the fire department's 450 paramedics who served 3.8 million people. The fire department's own psychologist found that "more than half the city's paramedics suffer burnout and emotional exhaustion.

About a third are dogged by extreme stress, the kind experienced by Vietnam vets who have seen and done too much. They complain of being overworked and undervalued."

The same article related our brother, paramedic John Smith, was diagnosed with "stress related hypertension. That's the diagnosis doctors give Smith after a series of tests. The doctors say they have good reason to suspect it's most likely job related."

The article stated, "There is a crisis among the 450 fire department paramedics. Short-staffed and forced to go on a record number of runs— roughly 200,000 in 1999— most are stretched so psychologically thin, it's not only hurting their job performance, it's damaging their lives."

The New York City Fire Department had roughly the same amount of paramedics, yet our call volume is more than 1.3 million calls a year. This is taxing on both paramedics as well as EMTs. The 1993 study by Drs. Jose Sanchez and Jack Kamerman has fallen on deaf ears. But EMS Office of Medical Management has never been noted to care about the crews who work under their license. Only one doctor did, Dr. Motley, and, needless to say, he was forced out.

In this cesspool of anti-paramedic/EMT environment, paramedic James Patrick "Bubba" Fallar reported to refresher. All morning, paramedic Tom Reynolds had noticed the usual cheerful, hearty leprechaun was subdued. His eyes were downcast and dull, the trademark impish twinkle in his eyes gone. During a break, whispering, he asked Tom to do a twelve-lead EKG. With trepidation, he confided having chest pains the night before. Tom, one astute paramedic, was so astonished by what the strip revealed and immediately called in one of the instructors. Like a midget volcano, conflicting emotions suddenly erupted in all their fury from Bubba against Tom and the staff. Though he knew the Street Saints had confirmed his greatest fear and were doing the right thing, James Patrick "Bubba" Fallar also loudly heard the death knell being rung for both the job he loved and, more importantly, his family's dreams.

A unit was called. They loaded then transported him to North Shore Hospital, Bubba violently protesting all the way. The reality was Tom and the instructors saved Bubba's life. But a dark, sinister, nightmarish reality also awaited him. After leaving the hospital, he followed orders and reported to BHS. The doctor finally looked up, "Oh, you're not a firefighter. Since you are a medic, even if it happened on a run you can forget LODI benefits," he said in a dismissive manner. Bubba walked out, devastated. His wife, daughters, all depended on him. At this point he could even lose his house. He applied for LODI as directed by the union representative. It was denied.

He had a non-typical angioplasty. Problems developed, requiring him to go for another operation. Several stents were placed inside his left anterior descending and right coronary artery. The operation was at Saint Francis Hospital, which is world-known for its coronary care.

During this period, he used all his vacation and sick time to get by. An emergency grant of ninety days was awarded, which he had to pay back, if he ran out of time. A light duty position was made for him. This is extremely rare, in fact almost unheard of, but people liked him, who wouldn't? It was in the Manhattan Borough Command (Enchanted Forest), answering phones, Bubba sweated, awaiting the results of a stress test as the darkening cloud of doom silently enveloped him. As the days turned into weeks, the clouds of despair turned to depression. The result would determine if he could go back to work as a paramedic or go to the unemployment line as a fired paramedic.

In November 2000, Bubba solemnly informed me he failed the stress test and had to go under the knife again, this time perhaps to have bypass surgery. "Jim, on this job, we are only one sickness away from bankruptcy." He mournfully told me, his voice cracking.

Firefighters spend less than four hours a day outside their houses. EMS crews spend all of their time inside of a bus. The bus was not made for sitting eight to sixteen hours a day. Yet, the crews are officially discouraged from sitting and eating like humans at their garages.

In fact, they do not get lunch or dinner breaks. EMS Administration went so far as to reprimand crews for going to the bathroom! Dispatches claimed they could "deny a facility (bathroom) request."

On October 23, 2000, The New York Post ran a story about twenty-eight-year-old Emma Christofferson, who died in London from what is called "Economy Class Syndrome" aboard a Quantus Air jet. She developed deep-vein thrombosis, a blood clot associated with long-distance flights. Think about being crammed in an economy class seat. There's not much more room in the buses, where we sit eight to sixteen hours a day.

Now let's compound this. How healthy do you think we are, sucking the fumes of our diesel buses? Diesel contains more than forty known harmful agents that produce cancer, asthma, and heart conditions. But more importantly, what is the response from doctors at BHS to injuries, or were Bubba and Denise just fluke cases?

Concerning the charlatan, jaded doctors at BHS, here is a personal experience. I had a foot problem from the boots issued so I went to see an orthopedic doctor named Mannon. Looking at the paper in front of her, she screamed at me, "You're not on my list. Go see a regular doctor!" When I attempted to explain the situation, namely that I was directed to see her, she would hear nothing of it and became more abusive. Totally frustrated,

I cut Dr. Mannon short. "Who the hell do you think you're talking to?" Having gained her attention I continued, "Now do you want to see this paper or not?"

"I don't want to see *your paper*," she snapped. "You are not on *my list!*"

"Fine," I raised my voice. "If you want to be a fuckin' idiot, so be it."

I walked down the hall where a firefighter on light duty had been handing out records.

"You know what this fuckin' idiot bitch said?" I asked. There was utter silence from all the firefighters seated in the chairs. Before he could respond, I continued.

"This fuckin' idiot bitch is yelling I'm not on her fuckin' list, so now I need to see a regular doctor. This is crap after being here since five thirty to sign in early and her showing up late!"

Before the firefighter could collect himself he had turned beet red; a firefighter sitting down said, "Here, brother, go in ahead of me."

Turning to thank him, guess who was there? You bet. You can also bet she stepped out of my way since Dr. Mannon was now on my shit list.

Later after seeing another doctor, I heard a firefighter on crutches complaining to all who would listen. The guy had one leg in a full cast—a cast, mind you.

His leg was broken the day before and he was ordered to see the "orthopedic doctor." This poor guy had followed orders and was now being thrown out, cast, crutches, and all because he wasn't . . . you guessed it, on *her list*.

Exiting the area, the firefighter who handed out the records had finally gained his composure. "You really shouldn't get so upset," he said meekly.

"Upset? Trust me, if I was upset you would definitely know it," I said.

"But here is a flash for all you firefighters." It became quiet again.

"You guys should learn from us paramedics and EMTs not to take any shit off these doctors. They may impress you folks, but they sure as shit do not impress us. They are here to serve us, not abuse us. Have a safe tour," I said, smiling, and walked out the door.

There are very few officers in EMS who deserve or even warrant respect.

Officers like Cathy Fuchs and Vinny Hanlon are hard to find, especially when Vinny still owes me close to $200.00. Yet with every generation, real heroes wearing the bars do surface and I've been privileged to serve with some.

There was a rookie EMT at the officer's station. The kid was so new he did not have any time accrued sick or vacation. One day, he approached the officer behind the desk and asked for a few days off. His father was having a heart operation. The officer passed the paperwork up to the chief. It was denied.

The kid reported into the station on the eve of his father's operation to find out the result of the officer's efforts. "Get in the command car," the officer behind the desk told him. A few minutes later, the lieutenant got behind the wheel and drove in silence to the borough office. Once there, he told the kid to follow him. The kid quaked in his pants as the officer entered the chief 's office. Standing in front of the pious, self-indulging chief, the young lieutenant started the one-way conversation. "Sir, perhaps you would like to explain to this man why he can't be at the hospital with his family while his father is having heart surgery? Furthermore, if he can't get the day, you can have my shield." Without allowing the flabbergasted chief time to respond, he pulled off his shield and threw it on the chief's desk. The man got the day.

The young officer's name was Joel Friedman.

He later became a deputy chief. Joel never forgot where he came from, his people, nor the public we serve. Joel would have crews take blood pressure readings to help educate the people of the community. He was very proactive.

But unfortunately, once he became deputy chief, the chiefs over him isolated both his contact with the troops, community, and ideas of creative change he would suggest.

To reiterate, good officers are hard to find but they are there. On the morning of January 22, 2001, as I entered my refresher class, I learned of the death of such an EMS officer. Lieutenant Barbara Poppo of Battalion Thirty-nine in Brooklyn was dead at age thirty-seven. After shoveling snow so her people would not get hurt, she reported not feeling well.

Crews offered to take her to Jamaica Hospital, but she wanted to go to Coney Island to be closer to home and her five-year-old daughter. Once at Coney Island, she went into cardiac arrest. The crews learned to expect the phone call each morning from five-year-old Colleen asking,

"Has my mommy gone home yet?"

On January 24, my last day of refresher, I worked on 64 Willie Three, to cover Battalion Thirty-nine's medic unit. The crews needed time to be together at the wake. If there was ever a doubt about the legacy of love this woman left, all you had to do was look at the swollen, reddened eyes of these street-tough crews. One crew member interviewed other members who knew the lieutenant. She wanted a collection of memories to give to Colleen. As she grows older, she can learn more about her mother.

I never had the pleasure of knowing or working with Barbara on a bus. She was a medic's medic, a Street Saint of Compassion. Barbara was unlike those who sold their souls to the Fire God to become rats in BITS. She remained true to the people and profession. Instead of tearing us down with amateur half-investigations and lies, Barbara lived the truth, recognizing the nobility of the EMTs and paramedics. She corrected from within and brought joy to the job. Officers like her are precious gifts.

Paramedic Eileen Dechon told one of my favorite stories. They had an elderly patient who screamed out, "I have Alzheimer's." Barbara patted her on the shoulder, calming her. In a soothing voice, she told the woman, "Don't worry, you'll forget about it."

She was indeed a street medic. The most important thing about her mom I want Colleen to remember is that paramedic Barbara Pappo, and later as Lieutenant Pappo, made a positive difference in people's lives. When she is old enough, Colleen will remember Mayor Giuliani and Fire Department Commissioner Thomas Von Essen speaking words of praise about her mom. Yet, these two attempted to destroy the job her mother loved. Unlike them, I want her to remember that her mom was a fighter and a gift to us. But most of all, she was someone who loved her daughter with all her heart.

On April 19, 2002, EMT Andre Lahens, age forty-seven, and his partner, EMT Michael Steffens, responded to a "cop shot." Their vehicle was struck by Sylvester Valle who sped through a stop sign and hit the crew broadside. Twenty-nine-year-old Mr. Valle had a blood alcohol level of .22, more than twice the legal limit. Andre, a former marine, ready to retire in a few months, was on a respirator because of massive head injury. His partner, Mike, would eventually leave the hospital in time to attend Andre's funeral. Andre was killed as he raced to save the life of a wounded police officer. In the end, the call was a prank, unfounded. Andre Lahens was buried on May 1, 2002, leaving a wife, Brenda, and two daughters, Afiya, fifteen, and Dara, thirteen.

On June 7, 2002, EMT Daniel E. Stewart, twenty-seven years old and a three-year veteran of Battalion Forty-four, took his own life. Reports stated he was overcome by months of sifting through debris and body parts at ground zero. Aside from working the first twelve days at the site, Danny went down on his off-duty days. He had gone for voluntary counseling once, but no one from the department bothered to follow up.

His passing came as a total shock to his brothers and sisters at Battalion Forty-four. Danny gave it all every day. In the end it killed him.

Think about Danny and the others next time you try to outrun an ambulance or give the finger to an "ambulance man."

On August 6, 2002, at 2:30 in the morning in Queens, EMT Wolf Louissaint's leg was pinned between the bus and a car driven by Jose Lopez. Family members of the patient Louissaint had been treating now unselfishly assisted the EMT. They valiantly chased and held Lopez, who attempted to flee the scene. Lopez was charged with driving while intoxicated. Once again, a Street Saint of Compassion, a true Currahee, baptized the streets of New York City with his blood.

James Patrick "Bubba" Fallar finally passed his stress test and returned to full duty after another bout with the charlatans at BHS. To his credit, he continued the fight and won. Currently, he is one of the newer instructors at the EMS Academy, and I'm happy to report the impish twinkle has returned to the potbellied paramedic leprechaun.

Post-911 Notes

January 17, 2006
New York Post
By Erica Martinez

"While NYPD Detective James Zadroga valiantly fought the Ground Zero illness that took his life last week, two city EMT's died in virtual anonymity of similar ailments. EMT Timothy Keller, 41 died June 23, 2005 and Felix Hernandez, 31, died October 23, 2005. Keller *"filed for workers' compensation-and was denied."* "Had the city not cut his medical benefits, he would have been able to pay for his medication," said his son. "To this day, Hernandez's family shies away from drawing attention to his heartbreaking death."

March 21, 2006
New York Post
By Erika Martinez

"An FDNY paramedic (Deborah Reeve)who died of lung cancer after working at Ground Zero was laid to rest in The Bronx yesterday…According to her family and friends she was *denied line-of-duty injury benefits and workers' compensation* for which she filed." Further into the article, "She was the third EMS worker to die in the past nine months of a possible 9/11 illness."

May 19, 2006
New York Post

City Wrong to $tiff Sick 9/11 Big: Mike

By Maggie Haberman and Carl Campanile

"The city's bid to deny a former Rudy Giuliani aide medical benefits for a suspected Ground Zero-related respiratory illness was "wrong," Mayor Bloomberg said yesterday.

"Rudy Washington is a really stand-up guy," Bloomberg said.

"The next thing I know was one of our lawyers, on a technicality, I thought, was trying to appeal his court decision and when I heard it, I thought it was wrong," Bloomberg added. "When I heard about it I just thought it was wrong and we changed it overnight."

Hours later, city Law Department official John Sweeney said, "The mayor has asked that there be a fair resolution to Mr. Washington's claim" - but said nothing about withdrawing the appeal.

Giuliani said yesterday he was pleased when he heard the city had backed off.

Lawyer David Worby, who represents 8,000 Ground Zero workers in a class-action suit, agreed.

"Why isn't Giuliani fighting for these people? The city is fighting them tooth and nail," he said.

Giuliani said it's impossible for him to judge other claims without knowing the specifics. "I know Rudy's," he said.

Just goes to show you who counts.

Nine

The Hoodlum Commissioner and
His Gestapo Rats

As stated in the previous chapter, the hope of a world-class School of Fire and Life required a proactive, creative administration to make it happen. For creativity to flourish, the environment must be conducive to the budding of diverse ideas with the noble acknowledgment of moving forward into the unknown together. This hope of mine was forever crushed when Mayor Giuliani allowed the Fire Commissioner to wantonly betray the Street Saints, firefighters, and citizens of New York by verbally acting like a third-class hoodlum on national television.

"Direct field observation of EMS units has identified certain practices with regard to cervical spine precautions and the application of cervical spine immobilization that need to be addressed."

Thus it was written on page two of the Continuing Medical Education News and Information, Volume 6, Issue 10, dated November 2000. This is a publication of the Office of Medical Affairs, Assistant Commissioner for Emergency Medicine, John J. Clair, and Lewis Marshall, M.D., J.D., Chairperson, Training and Testing Subcommittee.

The key words that jumped out were "Direct field observation of EMS units." This told me four things.

First, we were being observed and videotaped. Second, it was probably by BITS units. Third, if BITS management did not immediately correct a possible life-threatening mistake in the field, *they were knowingly assisting in hurting the patient.* BITS would be culpable in an injury case. A plaintiff armed with this information could claim, Res ipsa loquitor, the facts speak for themselves and win against the fire department.

Fourth, not taking immediate action to correct a life-threatening mistake leads to the conclusion that the real goal of the investigation was to get the dirt on the units so heat could be diverted from FD fire suppression units. I saw what was coming and mentioned it to other members at Battalion Twenty-six.

It did not take too long for the truth of my statement to come to light, but even I was shocked and awed at the prehistoric mentality and wannabee gangster image that would come from a NYC Commissioner. We had just received news that the union, led by President Pat Bahnken and Vice President Don Faeth, had secured for EMS a twenty-five-and-out pension for the members, signed by Governor Pataki. It had been a tough year for the union, which went from a scandal-ridden environment to a viable, resilient, fighting machine.

Pat had suffered personal humiliation when his drinking problem was disclosed. Rising above the mud slinging, Pat, being a man beyond his years, acknowledged the problem, stating he had been alcohol free for several years. This point somehow got lost between Giuliani and his lap dog. With Pat's leadership, we received what amounted to a three-quarter bill and twenty-five-year pension. If you were injured, the disability bill would finally be there for you. However, it would prove to be a horror to receive, short of being dead! Just ask paramedic Tom Reynolds.

Mayor Giuliani fought vigorously against the bill. He used his surrogate commissioner to run most of the interference. The Fire God also supported the for-profit ambulance company, MetroCare. The reason for this is obvious. First, MetroCare had helped Giuliani, thus the payback. Next, a point Local 2507 forgot to mention to the troops was that FDNY EMS was also for-profit, thanks to Giuliani, and finally for all its egotistical talk FDNY never could, never did and never will be able to provide enough crews, forget appropriate care for the people of New York City. This was due to an increasing bleed of experienced people fed up with mismanagement at best, criminal ineptness at worst.

In early spring 2000, the unheard-of happened as a twenty-five-foot rat was inflated in front of the commissioner's office at Puzzle Palace, 9 Metro Tech. This set the stage of revenge that occurred six days before Christmas 2000.

On December 19, 2000, Fire Commissioner Thomas Von Essen proclaimed to the media that nearly forty EMTs and paramedics, including four lieutenants, were bagged after a three-month investigation.

The investigation was sparked by an increase of several seconds in response times. He claimed to have spotted an increase of a "few seconds" in response times. Indeed an astute observation coming from a genius who couldn't notice a loss of over $34 million from accounting mismanagement.

This spike was questioned by the city council. City Council Speaker Peter Vallone was about to run for mayor and backed a bill to make EMS a uniformed service. The mayor's deceitful pettiness once again raised its ugly head, as he called out the Fire God. With much flair and little substance, one official stated, "They deserve to be fired. Thank God we did not have any fatalities, and no one was seriously hurt because of their negligence."

In the same article, the Daily News, December 19, 2000, stated, "According to a fire department document obtained by the Daily News, the findings of negligence came primarily against crews assigned to Brooklyn and Queens."

The Daily News cited a FD document, implying a _criminal investigation._

Yet neither the Fire God, nor BITS Assistant Commissioner Lai Sun Yee a.k.a. Dragon Lady, went to the police or even to a judge. Now a newspaper has access to a fire department document?

Between the fire commissioner and his lawyer, they never put together criminal with investigation. Yet the April 7, 1997 article previously mentioned stated, "The city Department of Investigations conducted a yearlong study of abuses in the system, but has refused to release its findings."

Seemed this refusal to release by Giuliani's DOI only pertained to firemen, not FD EMS. Gee, they claimed no knowledge when I asked concerning research for this book also. Does anyone see a pattern here concerning DOI, and FDNY?

Thomas Von Essen earned the nickname "Hoodlum Commissioner" with this statement to the press about what he'd do if he had found a crew member sleeping in a unit, "I would have taken a baseball bat to the front windshield."

Only a street punk would make such an irresponsible statement. But unlike the commissioner, a street punk would back it up with more than his mouth. Not even the commissioner's rank and file on the fireside liked or trusted him. All he had going for him is *his* Circle of Concern, First Deputy William M. Feehan, Chief of Department Peter J. Ganci, and his little rats, known as BITS.

His burning rage was spewed forth at those least likely in position to give him grief, yet even thru lava like flows of insults we remained unbowed.

Now that his fifteen seconds of fame was over, let's look at what type of investigation the "rats" accomplished and what the gestapo netted in the course of their investigations. Here are the secrets kept from the public we serve.

First, the inept morons fired an EMT who was not even at work. Next, they scored a direct hit on a unit sitting in the emergency bay at Kings County Hospital. Their correct 10-89 (street location) was in front of a bar, known for shootings. EMTs must be within four city blocks of the 10-89. The investigators stated the crew was in excess of that distance. The crew was falsified their signal.

The only problem was the county had two ways the unit could exit. If they went out the back way, the crew was

10-89. The new location was known and approved by the captain and borough EMS Chief.

These morons, I mean *investigators*, even hit Bellevue units. Lieutenant Vinny Hanlon was on the desk when 07Y1, my old unit, came into the garage to fuel on tour one. One of the medics stopped by for pleasantries, as his partner slept. After fueling, they got coffee and returned to the street location The investigators nailed Vinny for not realizing the crew was still 10-89 while fueling at the station. They also bagged the crew for being out of their 10-89.

Captain Stone's policy is to keep his 10-89 times good. My old unit, 07Y2, would remain 10-89, even at the garage with his blessing. Secondly, some people would call it pettiness, bagging either the crew members or Vinny. I would say it is pure bullshit like everything else BITS does to EMS crews. As usual, it was done in a half-assed manner, to get maximum photo (gee, what's a fireman without a camera?) publicity for the Hoodlum Commissioner. There was little substance to any of it.

To date, none of the crew received fines. The FD gestapo, BITS, forgot the 'I' in BITS stands for investigation. The morons could not even conduct a background investigation in a professional, logical manner.

April 15, 2007

The New York Post broke the story that FDNY firefighter Marc Von Essen son of the Hoodlum Commissioner Thomas Von Essen "Took a four year leave of absence to work with *Giuliani Partners*, yet is still entitled to a pension."

I ordered two pair of work pants on January 16, 2001 and was told they were out of stock, but I could come back to the Quarter Master in two days. Returned, still not in, so I stopped by on February 22 and was told they were doing inventory. "Your pants are in, but you can't have them now. They will be sent to your battalion on Monday."

On March 20, I was told, "Oh they will be sent out in two weeks." I bet a fireman will deliver them. These assholes took _three months to get me pants_, but the Fire God noted a drop in the response time of a few seconds. This is the crap I took working for the Fire Department of New York, and yes, they were delivered by a firefighter not on a fuckin little red fire truck!

Ten

Attack on America

On 9/11/01, I was traveling on a city bus to Battalion Twenty-six. Since being "detailed" to the South Bronx because I didn't play nice in the sandbox, I was given a breathtaking panoramic view each day.

To my left was the New York City skyline. I could see the Empire State Building and, further south, the World Trade Center. These concrete-and-steel giants reached brilliantly to the heavens. Aircraft soared from LaGuardia Airport, taking drowsy-eyed passengers on a magic carpet ride across this wonderful land known as America.

To my right, as we left the sleepy houses in Whitestone, Queens, we passed over Francis Lewis Park. Francis Lewis was an American teacher who was hung by the British during our War of Independence. The trees, bathed in shadows, gave silent testimony to his quiet determination and self-sacrifice. He was a teacher, not a soldier. Yet when he was called to make the ultimate sacrifice, he did—alone. He was a man of peace and courage. Little did I know that in several hours healers of peace and courage would join him on a bloody field of combat and I would be honored; by serving with them.

Below me was water of the East River. It playfully splashed upon a giant rock. Once when a dear friend of mine, Norma Iris Velez, was a little girl and came to visit me, we walked by the water. She saw the rock and thought it was an alligator. I smiled at the memory as I shifted my eyes to the real treat, the water. Today, it was like glass, with only a few ripples from a passing boat. How much nature reflects the human condition. My mind was at peace.

Ahead of me was the Bronx. There were no concrete-and-steel giants. On one side marshlands were being cleared and on the other the area was dotted with cottages. Here in Clason's Point, my grandfather owned a house many years ago. Looking toward Rosedale Avenue, I saw the Academy Gardens where I grew up. The red brick apartments climbed several stories.

When I arrived at Battalion Twenty-six, I checked in with Lieutenants Denise Werner and Giuseppi Lavore. I had been scheduled for overtime. As I stood in the office, I was told someone had crossed my name off the rundown and penciled in another paramedic's name. These people could not even keep simple rundown straight.

Lavore and Werner, who are rare breeds of outstanding officers, were upset over the rundown oversight. They wanted to do something to compensate me. I told them to forget it. Being senior to the medic in my slot and it was a beautiful day I opted to go home.

I enjoyed a nice breakfast and was on the computer when my cellular phone rang. "Jim, this is Tony from Croatia. I am calling to make sure you are okay." Tony and his family had befriended me when I was in Bosnia.

"Yeah, I'm fine. Why?"

"We are watching CNN and a plane just hit the World Trade Center," he yelled, as the connection got weaker.

"Have to run. Love ya," I said, as I disconnected.

I called the Bellevue EMS station.

Lieutenant Baskin said, "Get in here!"

I got into my uniform as I called a cab. Looking at my gas mask, I left it behind realizing this was a terrorist hit, until proven different. It was what I call a high-yield hit. The explosion temperatures would be high enough to evaporate whatever was aboard. In a low-yield hit, say in Grand Central Station, demolition would explode, yielding a lot of casualties, but not evaporating the people and building. The crews would assume the casualties were "contaminated" with an agent.

My plan was to head to the EMS Academy at Fort Totten. I knew an operation of this magnitude would require all our resources. When I got there, I leaped out of the cab and banged on the nearest bus (ambulance). The door opened and I climbed in as the convoy of ambulances pulled away with sirens wailing. Inside were paramedic instructors Rudy Havelka, Willie Silvestry, and others. As the ambulances screamed toward the Midtown Tunnel, one car actually tried to outrun us. Willie and Rudy yelled to the EMT up front to "Run the bastard off the road."

Suddenly, we could see the dense smoke blasting into the air. Even from our vantage point miles away, I could see the tragedy unfolding. The clear, powder blue sky was smudged black with death.

Some joked, others bitched that they had not brought their body protection armor with them. After combat in Vietnam, I recognized this is the way some people deal with fear. We all wanted to get there as soon as possible to assist the wounded and dying.

Silently I gazed out the window. Someone muttered, "It looks like war."

I replied, "This is war."

As we responded in, other units were on the scene, including my cousin Jerry of Rescue Three. Men from company after company climbed the stairs wearing their Scott Packs and bunker gear and carrying other equipment, including hoses—hoses made for water. In an aircraft fire, the fuel, JP4, requires foam. Water only spreads the burning fuel.

An eerie glow from the emergency lights illuminated the staircases. The light mixed with wisps of gray smoke. The air was becoming caustic. The firemen climbed, pushing past the evacuating, panic-stricken civilians.

The stairwells were choked with EMS crews, intermingled with the firefighters, climbing ever higher. The firefighters told civilians to return to their offices, everything would be okay.

Meanwhile, floors above them, the jet fuel was burning at more than two thousand degrees, melting the steel. The steel was the outer strength, supporting the building. Without this outer support, the building would collapse floor upon floor. Exhaustion was setting in as the crews were sweating, cursing, and getting tired. Each man, with his own hidden fears, continued on. EMS crews did not have breathing apparatus such as the Scott Packs, the fire retardant bunker gear, or the training, yet when the call came of a fireman down they responded.

Outside, EMS Deputy Chief Charlie Wells and Captain Mark Stone continued to order our EMTs and paramedics in—to their deaths. Paramedic, then EMT Byron Rodriquez was told to take his stretcher and equipment into the lobby of the first tower hit. Running through falling debris and bodies he told his partner who was at the front of the stretcher that if he felt Byron tug it meant stop. Captain Stone told Byron to "Stop sight seeing and get in there!" Once inside elevator's crashed to the ground floor exploding ejecting human torches into the lobby. Byron told Stone again they were too close.

More units responded in being told by EMS officers to park their buses in a neat line, directly under the burning building.

Finally by the saving grace an FDNY Battalion Chief told Stone, "Get your people out of here they have no protective gear!"

As Byron and other crews left DC Vallani told him to help on the MERV. Once again this EMS Brother of mine told Vallani the MERV was not in a safe location. At that moment they heard NYPD ESU crews near the waters edge using binoculars and bull horns said if anyone heard the following blast of a horn run for your lives. Suddenly it happened. Byron is credited with saving other EMT's, as well as a handicapped child that day. This man kept his head becoming a true leader when the inept EMS command was melting as fast as the steel. Years later when I had the pleasure of working with him as an outstanding Paramedic he told me how after 9-11 Captain Stone fearing he would say something thus endangering Stone's chances for becoming Deputy Chief told Byron, "I was doing as I was told." Yeah, didn't the Nazis say the same?

Prior to the collapse two lieutenants were relieved because they refused to send people to their deaths. Lieutenant E. "Pinkie" Albuerme, from Battalion Eight, Bellevue, was one of those heroes. He told the crews, "Don't listen to him. Get your gear and get out of here." A lot of people owe their lives to Pinkie.

EMS command violated procedures (EMSC OGP 106-06, section 5.3.9), which stated, "To ensure a prompt response to patients, EMS operations officers may be directed to establish a sector near the fire staging area. This sector will function as the Forward Triage Sector, and members will stand by at the location. Prior to establishing this sector, the EMS officers shall verify the location with the Fire Incident Commander, confirming that the environment is safe to enter."

It continues, "For example, during a high-rise fire, the Forward Triage Sector would be established below the fire. NOTE: An area unsafe for building occupants would not be considered appropriate for a Forward Triage Sector."

To reiterate, in the mid '90s, FDNY conducted a drill of a terrorist attack in the NYC subway system. It was such a success the Congress of the United States used the news videos to demonstrate to the rest of the country how _not to conduct an operation_ but it also showed our enemies how inept FDNY was then. Had they learned…afraid, not.

To add insult to injury, astoundingly, FDNY as well as the Battered Bastards (FD EMS) had practiced a mock drill one year earlier, "Plane into a high-rise building." During the exercise, EMS Command was ordered to pull their units back from the incident, fearing they were too close. On September 11, 2001, **_EMS Command would totally ignore lessons learned earlier_**, specifically placing crews directly in the kill zone.

More than one crew had gotten into trouble in earlier incidents when EMS chiefs directed crews to set up one to two floors below a fire floor in a burning building. EMS chiefs had violated their own rules for years, sending untrained, unequipped civilian EMTs and paramedics into burning structures to appease the fire department planners.

EMT Nelson Cintron and his partner Billy Truoccolo had responded to a fire in the South Bronx. The fire chief ordered them into the burning, smoke-filled building because he claimed to have a patient upstairs. Nelson refused; it was too dangerous. He asked for the patient to be brought out.

The response from the fire chief was, "I'm fucking ordering you to go in there!" Both crew members refused and offered to call a supervisor.

The response, "You better get me someone higher than a supervisor."

EMS Deputy Chief Fred Villani responded. The EMS crew stood by as firemen smashed the windows, venting the building. Clouds of white smoke and hot gases billowed skyward. Glass and window frames crashed to the street below like deadly missiles. The entrance was obscured by smoke. The Bravest ran more hoses into the small, water-soaked hallway.

Deputy Chief Villani declared the crew "should have entered, to see how bad it was." He reported to Chief Gabriel, another genius with no spine, who suggested the "crew lose a day's pay for refusing to go into the building." All of this was to satisfy the fire department battalion chief's ego, and by the way Chief Gabriel moved on to OMA (Office of Emergency Management).

September 11, 2001 was nothing new. Now, it would be up to EMS Deputy Chief Wells and Captain Stone to throw aside the established guidelines, safety of the crews and yes common sense. They wanted to look good for their Fire God master.

After the jet rocket hit the north tower of the World Trade Center, many people trapped inside, including Stephen L. Roach, called their loved ones. They called 911 begging to be rescued. Many were above the impact—cut off from the stairwells to safety, yet they would be murdered because of a decision based on pure FDNY ego, not good tactical decisions.

In the 1993 World Trade Center attack, it took more than ninety minutes for people to climb down the dimly lit stairs. Now in 2001 cut off, but very much alive, these victims searched for a way out. They smashed windows and waved pieces of clothing, to let rescuers know they were alive.

Mr. Roach was at his desk at Cantor Fitzgerald LP on the 105th floor. His first call was to his wife, telling her he loved her. In a second call, his wife heard the desperate shouts of her husband's co-workers, "Try the roof! Try the roof!"

Mr. Roach shouted, "There's no way out!"

They survived for an hour and twenty-eight minutes, languishing in the hope of being rescued. Slowly, they realized they would die horrifying and agonizing deaths. Floor by floor, the flames crept toward the roof, toward the humanity trapped. Floor, by floor the fire grew in its unquenchable hunger to consume all. Person by person watched, as a coworker, not yet overcome by the smoke, was incinerated in front of them. All they could do was waiting their turns.

NYPD pilot Greg Semendinger was outside, ready to execute the rescue. He received the fire department reports. There were several hundred people alive on the floors above the crash site. He and other helicopter pilots orbited and waited.

Unknown to the pilot, as well as the crews, the doors to the roof were sealed. This explained why no one was on the roof. The NYC Port Authority said the doors to high-rises were locked to prevent people from committing suicide by jumping to their deaths.

In a landmark piece of investigative reporting, reporters Scott J. Paltrow and Queena Sook Kim asked the hard questions about these needless deaths in The Wall

Street Journal, Tuesday, October 23, 2001. Unsatisfied with the Port Authority's answers, they sought the facts. Staff writers Michele McPhee and John Marzulli later independently confirmed their findings. In the New York Daily News, Wednesday, October 24, 2001, and the Wall Street Journal, it was reported that FDNY failed to use all the resources available. In fact, it contributed to the trapping, and subsequent murders, of more than seven hundred people. The New York Times would later report after an indebt study that number was to (1,974)one-thousand nine-hundred and seventy four .

Remember, the tower did not fall for an hour and twenty-eight minutes. The police helicopters were orbiting above within several minutes. FDNY chiefs were still seething from the initial World Trade Center explosion in 1993, when NYPD pilot Semendinger helped rescue twenty-eight people. At that time, the press played up the fact that a pregnant woman was removed to safety. In fact, I was there and felt it was an uncalled for rescue. Neither common sense nor facts ruled that day, but the rescue was a success.

The FDNY had been sharply criticized by Federal Emergency Management Agency (FEMA). Since the 1993 World Trade Center experience proved aviation rescues were successful, FEMA recommended FDNY aviation resources be incorporated into joint operations. FDNY blatantly ignored the suggestion to conduct joint drills with the police department—including the use of helicopters at the scene.

In 1988, as fire ravaged the First Interstate Bank, in helicopters were used to save eight people trapped above the fire. It happened in Los Angeles and the chief pilot, Paul Shakstad, was with the Los Angeles Fire Department's air operation division.

The FDNY plan was to use helicopters as a last resort—unless FDNY was flying *their* helicopters. Let's not forget the photo op. In their quest to control New York City, they tried, but failed to get their own aviation units.

A plan established that NYPD helicopters were to land at the nearest heliport awaiting fire department instructions. This meant they would wait for firefighters to get to the heliport then airlift the firefighters to the scene, to affect the rescue. In this scenario, FDNY's glory would be sustained, untainted by the police department, who were to "transport only". Remember my statement concerning the wall in the FDNY building at Ft. Totten pontificating how Engine so and so saved the patient then in small print in the corner it had, ambulance so and so transported the patient. Remember the two firefighters on TV stating "We save the patient and then the ambulance transports them to the hospital." Are we seeing a sick pattern here folks?

On 9/11, the NYPD pilots got on station within minutes of the initial aircraft hit and reported a smoke-free area on the tower. Now was the time to employ aviation in the rescue mission. Aside from the NYPD aviation unit there were other professional from the Army, and Coast Guard available.

At the moment of catastrophe, ego ruled FDNY decisions. FDNY was infuriated at the sight of the NYPD helicopters. They kept the aircrews in the dark as to the sealed doors. Not even the 1,974 dying souls could move them, or the hundreds of jumpers shame them to ask the choppers to land, so firefighters could open the doors. Thus Chief Ganci himself died in the collapse of a tower. I was there when they recovered his body but the fact remains he didn't employ all his resources. I'm sorry he died, but shit happens in war and folks we are at war so get over the "He's attacking a fallen brother" bullshit and examine the facts. The facts are once again FDNY failed under fire.

As far as the doors being "locked for security reasons with Fire Department approval," doesn't that hit the nail on the head as to where the blame sits? "Security reasons" are insufficient when they create life threatening problems which assist in murder. This _was not_ a sound tactical solution to save lives. _It was_ an ego saving solution which contributed to the murder. Furthermore, when the towers were designed, where was FDNY for the inspections? I keep hearing about fire prevention programs, well dah. We already know why

243

the doors were sealed but in the design phase didn't the architects *or FDNY* think about a disaster?

The second reason people died was the most obvious. FDNY had no workable plan to rescue those above the fire.

In response to the incriminating reports, Mayor Giuliani said, "I looked up at the building again and it seemed self-evident." Fire Department Chief of Department Peter Ganci had informed the mayor an air rescue was too risky. Yet pilots orbited, waiting for someone to come to the roof.

Later, Fire Commissioner Thomas Von Essen complained the newspaper stories were "hurtful." He suggested the reporters should have spoken to FDNY experts instead of individuals on the front line.

This makes no sense, unless you wanted to keep the Giuliani image intact. Individuals, not the experts, were the ones who made the difference.

It was the individual firefighters, police officers, EMTs, and paramedics who saved lives, not the paper-pushing administrative ass-wipe "experts." The *experts* of the fire department made a decision that assisted in the murder civilians, firefighters, police officers, paramedics and EMT's. Similar disastrous decisions would follow because of FDNY ego.

Inside the tower came the first violent shock wave of energy. The building shook and shuddered. The emergency lights went out. Fear overwhelmed. The heart-stopping fear you feel when you know, within your soul, you are about to die. Suddenly, a frantic call came across some of the firemen's radios to evacuate the building. Police Officers would later report telling firefighters to evacuate only to be told, "We don't take orders from cops!"

Fear turned to terror. A millisecond after the first call to evacuate came a blood-chilling scream, then silence. The acrid smoke filling the stairwells exploded.

More screams pierced the darkness. Suddenly, the darkness was illuminated with a light source—human torches several floors above. The stench of burning flesh filled the air. The agonizing screams would be the last sounds anyone in the hallway heard.

A rolling ball of fire and debris enveloped the crews as they attempted to outrun death. Stairwell after stairwell collapsed. Floor after floor disintegrated within the all-consuming fireball. Frantic screams were heard on our citywide frequency as EMS crews became trapped in the lobby and first floor of the collapsing, one-hundred-ten-story Tower One.

Captain Stone dashed from the building into the South Tower. Outside, some crews were in their ambulances, awaiting orders from EMS officers. In a flash, they were incinerated, never a trace to be found of them. Others managed to run for their lives, as the building pulverized everything below it.

Crews continued into the scene. The urgency of the situation was heard in the frantically screamed radio transmissions. The streets were clogged with a sea of humanity, running from the catastrophe. Going against this tide were the EMS units, who stood shoulder to shoulder with the police and firefighters.

One such crewmember was EMT Yamel Merino, who worked a MetroCare Basic unit. She pulled up with her partner. The acrid smoke burned their lungs. Outside was a living hell of falling steel and concrete, and screaming people. Bodies fell from the sky, like flaming cinders, crashing to the ground with sickening thuds. On impact, the body parts exploded, covering the area and crews with blood.

Yamel looked at her partner and said, "I'm scared. Before we get out, let's pray." They held hands and said a short prayer. Both EMTs exited the vehicle to join in the desperate dance of life. Yamel would become the eternal symbol of those who answered the call that day. She symbolized the best of the EMTs and paramedics of New York City during the darkest hour in our nation's history.

A despicable mayor and an ego-driven fire commissioner would ignore these heroes. These civilian employees, denied Uniform Status by a pathetic mayor, responded alongside the New York's Bravest (firefighters) and Finest (police officers). Looking death in the face and trusting in a loving God, Yamel stepped into the man-made holocaust. It was the last time she was seen alive. Much later, this single mother's burned body was found amidst the rubble of crushed dreams.

The building exploded. Each collapsing floor spewed glass, bodies, steel beams, concrete, and fire down on the rescuers. Paramedics Carlos Lillo and Richardo Quinn laid down their young lives that day. Carlos, whose wife worked in Tower One, would never know until after death that she escaped. He was last seen with tears running down his face, doing what paramedics and EMTs do, taking care of people.

In this inferno, people like EMTs Naomi Nacional, Ruben Rodriquez, and others continued to serve relentlessly.

A woman stood on a broken window ledge. Below she saw the burning building, further down complete mayhem. Choking from the acrid smoke, she looked back into the office. Co-workers huddled together in the corner. They had attempted to leave, but the stairwells were destroyed. Closing the door, they waited to be rescued. Now the door was jammed shut from the collapsing supports. Several men tried to pull it open, but due to the oven temperature heat, they burned their hands. The only light coming from her office was the cherry red glow of the door. Around the buckled frame, black, deadly, suffocating smoke was rushing into the office. Demonic red and orange flames voraciously licked the bottom of the door, craving the office's human content.

The woman could no longer see her co-workers, as the door glowed, slowly melting, but could hear them crying, amidst the muffled sirens of the rescue vehicles a lifetime below.

The fear of burning to death gripped her. She watched the grotesque scene outside. With a whoosh, several people passed the window as they plummeted to their deaths. Some screamed as they were blown out from the upper floors, their clothes and hair afire. Still others jumped silently, holding hands.

Above, a police helicopter hovered. The pilot had tried in vain to get close enough to extract people, even one person. He saw people in the windows waving, begging to be saved. But now his technology and skill proved impotent. No one was getting to the roof. He was reduced to hovering, praying, and being a silent witness to the living hell as tears ran down his cheeks. Tears that stained, and still at certain quiet moments run down our cheeks.Suddenly there was a loud crash as the door exploded, bringing the woman's attention back to the office. With a roar, a gigantic flame leaped into the office. She heard a co-worker's blood-chilling screams before it incinerated all. Now it was heading for her. Less than two seconds elapsed from the time the door blew open until the ball of fire approached the woman. In a heartbeat, she hurled herself out the window. Down she plunged, picking up speed. In the last one hundred feet, she watched the surreal scene below. Gaining speed, she approached the ground. Then there was darkness.

The jump from the sixtieth floor took only a few seconds. The woman's body exploded on impact. Her limbs were torn apart and her head separated. Bodily contents splattered other falling debris. Ruben narrowly missed being hit. He was soaked with blood as he continued to help others. A firefighter had not been so lucky. EMS frantically worked on him. One civilian ran up to a paramedic screaming "He needs help!" The man was carrying an amputated leg.

EMS command set the staging directly under the towering inferno. Paramedic Joseph Jefferson and his partner Rob Ruiz were near when suddenly, they were flagged down by a frantic firefighter. "Are you paramedics? Our brother is with the EMTs and they said they needed medics!"

Joe, a tall, reserved, gentle giant, got out of the bus and grabbed his equipment. He hurried behind the firefighter to the Basic unit, where the EMTs had the firefighter on the stretcher. Dr. Kelly, FDNY's Medical Director, said, "He needs to be intubated." Climbing into the unit, he felt for a pulse. "Doctor, he has no pulse," Joe reported in a calm voice, trying to convey a hint of reality. Still, the doctor feverishly administered useless CPR (cardiopulmonary resuscitation) to the dead firefighter still in his heavy bunker gear and no short board behind him.

Joe opened the airway in an attempt to intubate him, only to find a tide of blood, filling the dead firefighter's mouth. Dr. Kelly saw this and reached for the portable suction unit. With hands shaking she frantically splashed around in the dead man's mouth, yelling, "This is not working!" totally out of control. Joe gently, but firmly, directed that a finger be placed over the hole in the plastic tube, to create the positive pressure, which results in the suction. In her overwhelmed state she had forgotten even the most basic knowledge of patient evaluation. After several more pointless compressions she bolted from the ambulance, ordering Joe to transport the dead fireman to the hospital.

Looking at the dead firefighter, he attempted to put the laryngoscope blade into the firefighter's mouth, so he could place the tube into the trachea. Opening the airway, he saw the fire-fighter's face collapse before his eyes. The face now looked inhuman, almost like a plastic mask dissolving into a blob.

The ambulance was packed with firefighters. Joe gave his condolences, packed his equipment, and got out. Firefighters, of all people, entrusted their lives to us. They knew if there were a chance, we would go the extra mile.

As he walked to find his partner, Joe asked himself several questions. The firefighter was a black tag, meaning he was dead. Why was he being ordered to waste resources on a dead person? Why was the top doctor for the fire department breaking our orders for triage at a mass casualty incident (MCI)? Why the hell was she doing CPR on a dead person? The very people who trained and pontificated to us that they "were the doctors and you are paramedics" when faced with the reality paramedics and EMT's work in every day were out right failing when we needed them most.

Later, Joe and Rob's bus was totaled by the buildings collapse. Although both were wounded, they managed to save the lives of twenty people by evacuating them, before they returned to save more.

Deputy Chief Wells made another entrance on the scene and asked, "Who is the senior medic?" Everyone looked at Joe. "Get these people into the building. I'll be back in ten minutes." He walked away, leaving the crews to fend for their selves as the rest of the building came down.

Eighteen minutes later, the second kamikaze attack brought down the South Tower. With the twin towers down, burning Seven Tower was also in its final hours.

We stopped several blocks from ground zero, on the West Side Highway. There was complete chaos. I looked for an EMS officer but there was none to be found. I saw our FDNY EMS units, MetroCare (a private EMS service), City Wide, and Hatzolah (Jewish volunteers), as well as others. All were united in wanting to help, but no one was organizing them.

A police officer frantically asked, "Who's in charge?"

I looked around and said, "I am," then ordered the crews to set up a triage area to take care of the initial casualties. Then, maneuver them get for easy egress from the area. This would allow emergency units to move forward, yet allow our units to remove the casualties to the hospitals. Paramedic Hugo Sosa from Battalion 26 was instrumental in helping me accomplish this and conduct a fast resource count. The professionals from Hatzolah gratefully had responded in with extra gear so I knew we were in go shape.

Suddenly, the first patient made it to us. Realizing she was temporarily safe, the woman lost it. Having escaped the collapsing towers, she was overwhelmed psychologically by the ordeal. Screaming hysterically, she fell to the ground as EMTs rushed to her.

A cop asked, "What's going on?"

"She's not dealing with the stress very well," I said, still looking for an EMS officer.

The air was pungent with dust and the smell of death. The crews worked heroically as more patients, including firefighters, made it to our location. Critical patients were transported immediately. Non-critical injuries were dispatched by the busload to hospitals. The walking wounded and smoke inhalation injuries were packed into city MTA (mass transit) buses and taken to hospitals.

These EMTs and paramedics were awesome, each brother and sister whether Hatzolah, City Wide, Metro Care or FDNY EMS joining the Dance of Life working as one entity, healers.

Former paramedic Rob Rosenwald had worked at Bellevue Hospital before leaving FDNY EMS to work as an instructor at Bellevue's Emergency Institute. He walked up to me wearing scrubs. "Jim, I figured they had enough hands in the emergency room. Being a paramedic, I knew you could use me here." I was indeed glad to see Rob, but would expect no less of this brother.

As more patients arrived, I finally spotted EMS Captain Joe Apuzzo. He said we had to withdraw to Twenty-third Street and Chelsea Pier since there was a reported gas leak in this area. He turned and headed north to the staging area. Later, much later, it would be determined that WTC 7 where Giuliani's war bunker was located had a few problems. First, they had emergency fuel for vehicles both City and federal. Ok, you say, well not quite so fast. There were over 45,000 gallons of fuel stored in various parts of the building, and this was built over two Con Edison gigantic transformers, with gigantic diesel fuel tanks located on different floors with a natural gas line running through the whole shooting match! If that isn't enough, the electrical substation, supplied electrical power for all of lower Manhattan! All three components running through a building that OEM, FDNY, and the mayor expected to survive in. This was a disaster waiting to happen, but it even gets better. Did you know that the largest oil spill in American history was in and still is in Brooklyn, New York? In 1978 the Coast Guard reported to the State of New York that over 16 million gallons of oil had 'leaked' into Newtown Creek and most of it to this day remains under not only in the creek but in the soil and air! Of course it took the political pundits till 1990 to even slap the hands of Exon Mobile Oil Company. The point being, lower Manhattan is smaller than the area of the spill in Brooklyn. Green Point is the epic center of 'unknown' caused tumors, birth defects, cancers etc. The medical community has no explanation, but people blame their problems to the oil spill stating even the air quality has been effected. Thus, no one has reported the 'lost' oil from 7 WTC and I'm predicting another epic center of 'unknown' caused diseases in the years to come. Once again the politicians have failed to provide safety to its citizens or hold anyone accountable. Concerning the Federal Government let us not forget the EPA lies.

I went from one vehicle to another, ordering the crews to withdraw and, most importantly, informing them why. After combat in Vietnam and working under fire in Bosnia, I knew, when in a fight for life, you need not explain everything for people to respond. But if you can spare a second to keep them informed, it improves the team effort.

The highway was covered two inches of white cinders. It was difficult to breathe with the ash falling. I cursed myself for not bringing my personal gas mask as my lungs burned.

Then I saw Captain Stone standing alone. He looked at me, speaking about how he had cheated death. As Tower One fell, he ran to the second building. When Tower Two collapsed, he was struck by wreckage being dragged to safety by two of the Bravest.

"We lost people, Jim," he mournfully uttered. I guess he was looking for sympathy. Yes I was glad he was alive but sympathy...

Looking him straight in the eyes. "What did I tell you? What the fuck did I tell you?"

He couldn't answer me because we both knew the truth. Our people should have never been that close. But EMS command, including Captain Mark Stone, was so far up the fire department's ass, they sacrificed our people to make points.

Firemen fight fires, but there was no excuse for EMS Command not to expect terrorists. A plane hitting the World Trade Center on a clear day was as red a flag as you could expect. There was simply no excuse to place crews in harm's way. No excuse at all. I walked away my boots sinking into the thick ash as he nursed his injured shoulder.

As we pulled back on the West Side Highway, I saw a sea of exhausted firefighters, police officers, and EMS crews assisting the wounded and dying. I loudly suggested we walk by the water, away from the buildings. First we were a channeled element with the water to our left and buildings to our right. I expected secondary hits from the terrorists because that's what I would have done. I heard a firefighter repeat the same thing to several of his men, as they staggered after us.

"Good to hear somebody is thinking the same way," I said, looking into his tear-soaked, dirty face. He nodded the same look on other faces—the thousand- yard stare anyone in combat has seen it, worn it. Their souls were filled with a horror and sadness of overwhelming magnitude. It was reflected in empty eyes.

Among the heroes of New York, the thousand-yard stare was showing its ugly head, yet the fight for life had just begun.

Behind us, as the smoke got thicker, the breadth of the horror set in. The terrorists had done their homework since the last bombing. Ramzi Yousef, the reported mastermind of the 1993 bombing, had crippled the tower, but had not taken it down. I had no doubt then, or now, Osama bin Laden was behind both hits.

The terrorists had done their homework well, but not good enough. They declared war on America in New York

City, the greatest city on earth. Here in Manhattan, we are all Americans, from immigrant stock. We are immigrants from every culture, every religion on earth. New York City epitomized America. The terrorists had made a fatal error; firefighters, EMTs, paramedics, police officers, and Native American iron workers galvanized into one American family which wouldn't break.

One of the heroes that day was EMT Thomas Monahan. He decided to stick by my side and help. At this point we needed to secure some water and I had to leave some. When nature calls, a kid has to do what a kid has to do. So we broke away from the human tide and entered a college. As Tom went to get some water, I walked into the open bathroom. I froze. Several feet away from the wall stood a lone, oversized rucksack.

I approached it and noticed there were locks on it. With the proximity to the wall, I figured it was a bomb, a secondary devise. Hell this is what I'd do. Looking around and the bathroom appeared empty. Bomb or no bomb, I had to piss. If I were going to die, at least I wouldn't have to worry about my body being found with urine stains on my pants, if they recovered my body at all.

I heard a noise to my left and approached the stall, ready to kill the terrorist. I swung into the stall, and saw a man sitting on the toilet. He curled up, screaming.

"Who the fuck are you, asshole?" I screamed. The guy told me his name. He was a reporter. "Is that your fuckin' bag?" I screamed.

"Yes," he said, cowering.

"You're a real fuckin asshole leaving that alone. Get the fuck up and clear the fuckin' building. Now," I screamed. He pulled up his pants, grabbing the rucksack as he ran for the door.

Relieving myself in peace I stood there, a smile came across my face. I'd chased the reporter out of the bathroom without giving him time to wipe his liberal ass.

Outside, I caught up with Tommy and we rejoined the flood of emergency crews departing the area. I noticed an

EMS officer and asked the location of the MERV (Manned Emergency Response Vehicle). The MERV is like a large Coca-Cola truck, holding four stretchers and a lot of equipment.

"Over there, on the other side of the gas leak," was his response.

"Did anyone warn them?" I asked.

"Crews will get the word."

"That's not what I asked. Did anyone physically get there to warn them?" I asked.

"No," came a curt reply.

"Fuck this," I said.

"Where are you going?" asked Tommy.

"To get word to the crews these assholes are writing off."

"I'm with you," he said. Looking at the dogged determination in his eyes, I knew there was no point in arguing with him.

"Let's do it, brother," I said as we headed for ground zero and the unknown.

We proceeded down West Street, the air got thicker with white powder. It was at least two inches thick and still falling. For protection, we used rags over our noses and mouths, as we cut across Warren Street, heading east, then south toward the towers at Greenwich Street. As we walked, coughing our burning, acrid lungs out, and with our eyes tearing, we informed EMS crews still working on patients, FDNY, NYPD, and civilians to withdraw. We told them the triage area was set up at Twenty-third Street and Chelsea Pier.

Later, I learned Dr. Richardson did a great job at the triage area. He worked with the crews and let the doctors know who was in charge not about to waste the talents of our paramedics. He put one paramedic in charge of four tables, with the doctors realizing they, the doctors, were out of their element. He knew how to maximize his most precious resource, the paramedics.

Tom had split to warn several crews on the next block. I finally spotted a lone EMS unit and flagged it down. Manning the vehicle were EMTs Nicole Ferrell and Paul Alvarez. A lieutenant and chief had ordered them to go to the corner of Barclay and Greenwich Streets and wait. The chief said he would "be back in ten minutes."

"Is anyone there now?" I asked.

"Yeah, the chief should be there," Nicole said adamantly.

They pulled down the block after a heated discussion with a volunteer fireman trying to be a boss. A white cloud of dust climbed skyward from the tires. The scene looked like Pompeii after Mount Vesuvius erupted. I followed them on foot, my lungs burning. No point in riding. I could see more walking.

Once there, I listened as the crew told me they had been in the building with the firemen rescuing and evacuating people.

"They need us here to help with the wounded."

As I stood next to the bus, looking and listening to these two precious heroes, I realized that Seven Tower looked, felt, and smelled like it was coming down. Aside from being too close, the asshole chief was not coming back. He'd save his own ass while abandoning these people.

We waited several more minutes and a Hatzolah ambulance pulled up. I decided to move, telling both units to load everything that was set up on the ground into the buses. We would leapfrog back using buildings as protection. If we found wounded, we'd put them into the buses. Both crews listened and we started our retrograde movement.

We moved back till we got around Chambers Street. Once there, we headed toward the water and West Street, spotting an exhausted NYPD ESU (Emergency Service Unit) police officer staggering. As Tommy and I clutched him, he asked, "Is that you, Schrang?"

"Yeah." He was an EMT in the early days remembering me from King's County in Brooklyn. As I held him, Tommy got my heroes, EMTs Ferrell and Alvarez. He would be in good hands with them.

Tom and I hooked up with other FD EMS voluntary and private ambulances when I saw a welcome sight. Captain Jo Ann McFarland had taken command and wanted me to assist her. Finally, someone was doing the right thing.

I met other EMTs who were at the stage of physical collapse. Most were beat up, but not one, not one was about to leave the scene.

EMS Deputy Chief John McFarland met us. He was ordered to go into ground zero and give his evaluation. He asked if I wanted to go back in. Ha, such a foolish question from a mere mortal. As I started out with the chief, Tommy asked where I was going. The three of us left and walked into the blinding, enveloping cloud of white powder.

I had been an army paratrooper in Vietnam with the Screaming Eagles and had traveled to Bosnia in the early nineties to help the Muslims, Croats, and Serbs during their genocidal conflict. But this sight was numbing, surreal. The white ash was turning a dirty gray and covering everything. Before us was mangled wreckage of buildings. Fire trucks had snapped in half, like matchbox toys. Body parts no longer bled red, as they became covered in ash and congealed to gooey remains.

Burned and crushed ambulances stood as testaments to the fury and terror of the attack. In the twisted wreckage of steel and concrete, I caught a glimpse of a burned EMS helmet. What happened to the owner? How much of the white ash was from the victims who were incinerated?

I later learned the ash contained far more than 1,974 cremated people left by FDNY to die alone above the fire.

I had to remind myself to remain focused. There would be a lifetime for these thoughts and insights to surface. From within the twisted carnage, the fires of humanity still burned, thus I had to remain focused on the mission.

We stood outside Three World Trade Center. Searing flames scorched the ground. Plumes of orange flames licked the sky, as if hungry for more death. Police and fire department resources started to get organized. Some windows were blown out, while others sat with jagged glass. Three floors above on the outside, a sharp sheet of metal, six by eight feet, hung precariously from the eastern wall. The cataclysmic explosion had embedded the sheet into the building.

To our south, the North Bridge had collapsed across the highway, crushing cars and possibly trapping people. The brute force of the exploding buildings twisted the steel beams like licorice sticks.

This is where I found my cousin Jerry's truck. All night long I walked back to the truck, hoping against hope he would return for equipment. Perhaps someone would know something about his fate. No one came. No one knew. In my heart, I did.

As the firefighters watered down the fires, a river of gray black mud formed at our feet. At this point neither our radios, nor my cell phone, were working. Deputy Chief McFarland attempted repeatedly to use the radio.

We weren't the only ones who had lost communications. FDNY "experts" had placed all their aerials and repeaters on the tower. When that went down, so did communications. Worse yet, all of the firehouses in lower Manhattan lost power and communications.

According to an article by William Van Auken of The Chief, entitled, "Whistleblower Suit," more happened that day. The computer system was supposed to continue operating with battery backup, but the batteries were either missing or not functioning.

John J. Fabbricante, a twenty-year city employee, transferred to the fire department when the EMS/FD merger took place. He reported startling facts in a lawsuit.

Starting in the mid-nineties, FDNY dropped its maintenance program for the emergency backup power units in the city's firehouses. The power units became useless pieces of metal. The firehouses desperately needed commercial generators. After he found an FD EMS station still without adequate power, Mr. Fabbricante brought his concerns to the city's <u>Department of Investigation (DOI)</u>. For his trouble, his "confidential" report was *leaked* and he was branded a rat by both FDNY management and Local Three, (Gee doesn't this sound familiar?) He was harassed, received death threats, rubber rats, and the like. This was before the World Trade Center catastrophe.

FDNY retaliated against people who tried to do what was right. Instead of being concerned with emergency communication equipment and power supplies, FDNY was more concerned with selling sweatshirts at the Fire Zone Museum. The results of their indifference came home to roost on 9/11.

As I stood at Tower Three, I wondered why no one in EMS command had a satellite phone. There was just no excuse for these bumbling idiots.

In the crowd was Dr. Dario Gonzalez, our Medical Director. He had gone to Oklahoma City after the fact and come back with war stories of being traumatized—without ever seeing a body. Now he was a useless, impotent observer. Not once did he ask how we were or how many wounded and missing we had. Not once did he think to ask what medical supplies we needed. He wasn't even concerned with a triage area. All he cared about was standing with the fire department brass.

Deputy Chief McFarland asked me to conduct a reconnaissance of the area and set up a forward triage area. As an afterthought, Dr. Gonzalez, said, "Take those doctors with you." He never looked me in the eyes. He was punching the clock as an observer. I, too, wanted to punch some-one's clock. As I walked away, I knew Gonzalez would be back with more war stories. But he realized I knew the truth.

Several volunteers stood by an abandoned Saint Vincent's ambulance. I grabbed some doctors and had them strip the vehicle for supplies.

Then we headed west. Walking up Vessey Street, we came to North End Avenue and made a right. The street ran north and south. To the south, one block down was a dead end. This was a good location for setting up the MERV. To the north was a clear run to Chambers Street. With its many intersections, we could bring in supplies and evacuate the dead and wounded. I wanted the resources on North End Avenue so the existing buildings could provide protection for the crews. Seven World Trade Center was burning and in its final death throes. It was just a matter of time before it came down. During my reconnaissance, I did a debris analysis of the other buildings. This was knowledge gained in the military, vital information that would give me an idea of what to expect when WTC 7 came down and how to protect both the crews and causalities.

It was a sure bet a lot of debris would fly up Vessey Street, thus the priority was to keep the crews and our scant resources protected. I gave directions to Tommy and he took the doctors and other remnants of the crews and started to set up. I returned to Deputy Chief McFarland and gave my report. Twice I returned to see how Tommy was doing, only to find everything moved onto Vessey Street.

"Tom, what the fuck?" I asked the first time.

"I set up like you said, but some captain came by and told me to change it."

"Well, move them back," I said, as I walked off. The second time I told him, "When this ass wipe shows up, send him to me."

Later I learned it was Captain Pineda from the EMS Academy. Again, no common sense; I informed the chief that I reset the group for the third time. He seemed pleased, but was really getting upset. The chief and I had been friends for years so I reminded him we were at war.

"Sir, a firefight is nothing more than organized confusion. So go with the flow."

The radio was now working, but there was no discipline from the captains and chiefs who were yelling incoherently. Really, would you expect anything different?

The chief asked me to get a crew member to bring an ambulance to serve as the morgue truck from Captain McFarland's position. This seemed like a waste of resources, especially at that location. Initially, he wanted to pull a unit in from my staging area on North End Avenue, but the crews wisely refused.

One problem was the crew would have to run down Vessey over the fire department hoses. The Bravest were fighting fires and racing the clock. The sooner the fires were out the sooner rescue could begin. The longer the fires burned, the longer they were consuming the life-sustaining oxygen of those trapped.

On Vessey, the bus would get stuck in the mud, creating more problems for the Bravest. The area was littered enough with the skeletal remains of ambulances, fire trucks, and humans. That staging area would be a waste of scant resources and, with Tower Seven burning, it would endanger the crews. When I told him of the crew's decision, the chief was enraged.

I trudged through the mud to Captain McFarland's location. She said a unit was on the way. That meant the unit was traveling on the dividing island that runs on West Street, one building away from Tower Seven. This made sense as far as helping stay clear of the hoses, but still a waste of resources.

Standing next to a police officer, I looked down and noticed a weapon on the ground. Then I inspected the area closely and found a hand. EMTs helped clear the area and we found the body. It was a Port Authority police officer. Like a small nuclear explosion, the force had blown him out of the building and across the highway. He was found buried in the mud and ash, more than a city block away from his office. While the people dug out the dead officer, another EMT crew member carried a wounded civilian.

A police chief, seeing an open ambulance, directed the crew to place the civilian in it. Deputy Chief McFarland went ballistic and screamed, "That's a morgue vehicle."

The bickering continued back and forth, the two ranking officers carrying on like children. Ignoring the tantrum, I walked over and asked about the civilian's injuries. His arm and leg were hurt, but he could walk. I directed the crew to walk the man back to Captain McFarland's position.

Suddenly a hush came over the crowd as all heads turned toward the observers, Dr. Gonzalez and the fire brass. They had located Chief of Fire Department Peter Ganci's body. This was why the chief wanted a morgue vehicle. Even now, politics were being played.

"I need that vehicle now!" Deputy Chief McFarland yelled at me.

"Fuck the dead," finally realizing what this was all about. I yelled. "This is fuckin' war! Fuck the dead!

Line them and the pieces up on the fuckin' sidewalk. Think about the safety of your crews. Let's fight like hell for those still trapped and alive."

He stormed off.

The crew of the ambulance approached. "We have to see the chief," one of them said with panicking apprehension in his voice.

"What's wrong?" I asked.

"The bus is dead. It won't start."

"Listen, you guys go up the block and team up with the other crews. Leave the keys in the bus. I'll tell the chief." After witnessing the tantrum and screaming, this crew did not need to be told twice.

I walked over to Deputy Chief McFarland. "I got some bad news for you John."

Relatively calm now, he asked, "What is it?"

"Your bus, the morgue, is dead." He exploded as I turned and walked away. It was clear Deputy Chief McFarland was not handling the stress very well. And, once again, good old EMS had been penny-wise and dollar-foolish bit them in the ass having installed the buses with the cheapest batteries.

I walked from one abandoned vehicle to the next, retrieving equipment. It was haunting, just like Vietnam. I wondered what happened to the crews.

Firefighters were making some headway in suppressing the fires in front of Three World Trade Center.

Suddenly everyone froze. The sound was unmistakable. It was jet engines!

The bastards are going to hit another building! As long as I live, I will never forget what happened next. Firefighters, police officers, EMS, and construction workers looked skyward into the haze. Then, silently, it happened. We _were not_ leaving this hallowed ground.

They could hit us again, but, by God, we were not leaving! Forming an unspoken, sacred human shield around our fallen, we waited, unwavering. Each of us dug deep, conquering our own fears, each mustering our resolve as American brothers and sisters. This was our, sacred ground, these dead civilians, firefighters, cops, EMT's and paramedics were our brothers and sisters, and this was our fuckin fight!

The whine grew louder, but the silence among us was deafening as creation waited for one of us to break the unspoken oath and allow fear to rule. Each of us had made our decision. It was as if the souls of the murdered watched acknowledging our feeble act of love. The Creator's hand gently swept across the area, suddenly the wind shifted, and the haze cleared. Flying above was an F-15 Eagle. Everyone let out a collective sigh of relief as the pilot came in again. We had air cover. Even the doubters could not ignore the fact, we were at war.

Meanwhile, remnants of EMS command tried for some semblance of order. As Deputy Chief McFarland made his attempt, Deputy Chief J.P. Martin requested HAZMAT (Hazardous Materials) units from the staging area at Twenty-third Street and Chelsea Pier.

Division Six Commander Frances Pascale was heard reportedly muttering, "I'm not sending anyone else. I've lost too many people. I'm not sending one person. I've lost too many people." Deputy Chief Martin pleaded with the shocked chief, to no avail.

Because of their deployment, the HAZMAT crews were so blocked in they were a useless resource. Deputy

Chief Martin worked with whatever he could get his hands on as his efforts started to materialize into progress.

Deputy Chief McFarland wanted to set up the forward triage in Three World Trade Center. Earlier in the day it had been abandoned, for safety concerns. Now he was ordering people back in.

Lieutenant Barry Travis, my former partner at King's County, refused to go or send people there. He just flat-out refused because the building was too close to Seven Tower.

In front of everyone, the chief screamed he was in charge and relieved Barry of duty. I intervened, reminding the chief of Sun Tzu's words, "The emotional warrior never wins."

"Okay," Barry said calmly. "Where do you want me to go?"

The chief responded, "I don't care if you jump in the river." He turned, eyes glaring, and ordered people back to the building. Barry stood there.

"Can't take you anywhere, can I?" I said, eliciting a smile from him.

This is what happens when the pencil-pushing ass wipes of EMS command are more concerned about teaching officers to write CDs, than educating them about leadership skills. I knew John McFarland was better than this. If he weren't, I sure as hell would not be with him now, or be his friend. But stress under fire can be a frightening, unyielding master.

Lieutenant Travis stayed in another area needing his help. After witnessing McFarland's tirade and insulting remarks, several crews and doctors asked me what I wanted them to do.

I replied, "Hey, I'm just a paramedic. What do I know? He is the chief."

A female Asian doctor from Flushing Hospital responded, "No, you are more than that." I smiled. She had been great all day. It was an honor to be with her.

"What are you going to do?" she asked.

"I'm going to watch the equipment for a few minutes," I said.

The crews followed the chief down the street. Suddenly at about 5:20 PM there was a scream as Seven Tower disintegrated with a dull roar. A cloud of deadly smoke and debris started to follow the people, who were now running toward us.

"Get in the buses and button them up!" I yelled.

People piled into the buses, slamming the doors behind them as the cloud approached. The EMS crews, with Deputy Chief McFarland in the lead, ran for cover. I gingerly stepped to the side of the building till the storm subsided. None of our crews were hurt or buses damaged. The surrounding buildings saved them. I looked at Lieutenant Travis. "Well, Barry, I guess it's safe to go into Three Trade now." He smiled.

Later that day, well over eight hours after the collapse, a Port Authority police officer was found alive. The cop was ambulatory as he emerged.

The crews gave him a round of applause. He was physically intact, but mentally, well, brother officers took his weapon away. They escorted him to EMTs in my triage area.

As dusk set in, I suggested to the chief that he should think about relief for the crews and CISM (Critical Incident Stress Management) teams.

I walked into Chevy's Fresh Mexican Restaurant. It was filled with firemen and construction workers. The proprietor kept putting out food. Anything we wanted was free, from food to sodas to liquor. The gentleman was great to all of us. Tommy and I sat at the bar, eating and drinking soda. I'd wait till I left this hell for my beer.

At dusk, the unreal landscape turned into Hades. Harsh white lights cut through the gray white smoke. Fires illuminated the grotesque, tangled steel. Orange flames lapped at the Bravest, as they continued to fight. The sight was burned into my very soul that night. EMTs wore glowing bands on their helmets. These were used for identification, since they did not give enough light for anything else. The bands helped keep tabs on people working away from the searchlights.

Police ESU crews wore gas masks as they dug deeper into the debris.

Buried under tons of rubble, a fireman lay pinned between slabs of concrete and debris. As he became conscious, he realized his body was unable to move. He attempted to move his head, but it was wedged between his helmet and broken Scott Pack face shield. His stomach hurt. The rush of air through his broken faceplate had awakened him. Through the crack in the debris above, he saw light. He figured it came from a lantern. When he called out, no one responded. With energy waning, he felt the cool air on his blood-soaked face. The air also blew the concrete powder; some of it clung to his face.

Suddenly there was a shift of debris in front of him. With the shift, the light was gone. Mustering all his strength, he cried out again. In the darkness he felt alone and frightened; resting his head, he softly cried. Only the sound of the oxygen kept him company. Suddenly the beeper blared as his heart raced, realizing the tank was almost out of oxygen.

Then there was silence. With the oxygen flow gone, all he could smell was the concrete and the heat from raging fires. The fumes were starting to get to him as he choked, gasping for air. If we listened closely that night, we could hear the beepers go off—the sounds of Scott Packs signaling the missing firemen were out of oxygen.

Everyone tried to locate the sounds, before the silence. Dead silence. Looking into the eyes of the Bravest, I understood. The silence drove another stake into their hearts, marking another brother gone forever.

With dogged determination, they, along with everyone else, worked on as the sun set and the fires grew.

At other times we heard gunshots. At first we figured it was from trapped police officers signaling with their weapons. Later, we learned the truth. The rounds were cooking off in the fires, as the officers' bodies burned.

Needing more supplies, I made my way to the MERV located in Captain McFarland's sector. There I found Reggie Jenkins, the EMT MERV operator. The vehicle's drug bags were gone, stripped from the vehicle in the initial minutes of the day. There had been no discipline; it was an open house to grab and run. This was not the way to manage resources. I did find an intubation kit and some fluids.

Back at Three World Trade Center, I saw it had been transformed into a forward triage and a morgue area. Bodies, as well as pieces of bodies, were being recovered. A doctor came over, complaining that he did not have an intubation set, as he eyed mine.

"Well, doctor, if the patient has to be tubed between the pile and where I'm standing, he's dead. If, on the other hand, he gets to you breathing, but needs to intubated—"

Cutting me off, he said, "Then we doctors will do it." Laying out his turf, this guy had neither grace nor wisdom.

"Wrong, sir. If he gets to you and needs to be intubated, you sir will be knocked on your ass as a NYC paramedic tubes him."

Two exhausted paramedics standing nearby smiled. The doctor knew the turf was ours. This was our arena. We would accept all the help we could get, but it would be ours to accept. Looking at me, then at the two medics, he said, "Okay," and walked into oblivion.

Replacements came and I had two fully equipped paramedic units from St. Vincent's Hospital and new EMTs from the academy. These kids looked so clean, so new, and so scared. Paramedic Joe Hodak was sent back to the academy with others who had labored all day. No one wanted to leave.

One of the EMS lieutenants came up to me, "Okay. You're out of here."

I looked at him. "Fuck you."

"What did you say?"

"Fuck you. I'm with Chief McFarland, and friends do not leave friends."

"Oh, I didn't know," he said. I looked at this moron, with his EMS management mentality that got our people murdered.

"Then ask," I said, walking away.

Chief McFarland was with his wife, Jo Ann, when I caught up with them. The three of us hobbled over to a chair so Jo Ann could sit. She had previously hurt her back.

"You know, all we need now is some rousing Spirit of 1776 patriotic music, the way the three of us are hobbling here." They chuckled.

After Jo Ann left to go home, John sat down and asked me to take his pulse. It was irregular so I called over a team of medics. The monitor showed some elevations in a few of the leads as well for his blood pressure.

He admitted to having some chest tightness.

"You think?" I asked.

"How's it look?" he asked, concerned.

I looked at the initial twelve lead. "Piece of cake, let's work him."

He focused directly at me, not talking to the medics.

"How am I doing?" His voice was filled with more concern.

"Well, shit head," that got him to laugh, "You would not listen to me when I told you about the emotional warrior never winning, right?"

John nodded and the two medics were oblivious to what I was saying. "Thus the results of those uncontrolled emotions have manifested themselves in elevations in the leads. No big deal. Just lessons, we can fix."

After ministering with the IV, aspirin, and nitroglycerin, we took him to the bus on the stretcher.

It was past midnight and Vessey Street was a nightmare. It was choked with shells of abandoned vehicles, fire hoses, spent equipment, mud, and white ash. Tired crew members plopped down wherever there was dry ground, awaiting their turns to work while the fires continued to burn. It would later be established that the federal as well as local governments lied concerning the air quality we were

267

breathing, yet to date I've yet to see a study of the environmental impact the diesel fuel alone from WTC 7 has caused. Mind you, only a microcosm of it has been recovered.

In the bus, John asked me to hop out at the EMS command post to tell Jo Ann what happened. Fire department vehicles were everywhere, no semblance of order, a real cluster. I spotted the Bellevue MERV. That wasn't the command center so I was sent from one location to another looking for the EMS command post. Finally, in frustration, I yelled, "Where the fuck is Chief McCracken?"

One of the EMTs looked at me with the thousand-yard stare.

"Evidently you didn't look far enough up (FDNY Commissioner) Von Essen's ass." That was the first time I really laughed all day.

I found the bus and on the way to St. Vincent's told John that Jo Ann had gone home. After arriving in the emergency room, John was evaluated and sent upstairs. John and I watched the TV in the room while we waited for Jo Ann.

A fireman, detailed to the hospital as a member of the Help Team, walked by. If a fireman needs something, the Help Team members assist him. He saw me slumped, exhausted in my dirt-covered uniform in a chair.

"Oh, you a fireman?"

I looked at him wearily, "No, paramedic."

"Oh," he said, indicating my unimportance to him. "What about him?" pointing to John.

"He's a chief," I said, already knowing where this was going.

"Oh," he said with anticipation in his voice. "An FD battalion chief?"

Both John and I looked at him. "No, an EMS chief."

"Oh," he turned and walked out the door. He didn't even so much as ask what happened or "how do you feel," or say "I hope you feel better."

I looked at John. "Guess we will always be bastard children to this department, huh?"

John laughed. "Yeah, you're right about that."

Much later, Jo Ann showed up. After a visit and being satisfied John was okay, she drove me home. The roads were open only to PD, FD, and EMS, the Trinity of Emergency Service.

On the way home across the bridge, I looked out over lower Manhattan. Against the darkness and the billowing smoke in the harbor stood The Lady, The Statue of Liberty. There she was with her light of freedom burning brightly. It seared through the man-made haze of insanity. Unyielding, the torch of love burned even brighter this night. The flames of freedom and hope were fed by the actions of the NYC Police Department, Port Authority, firefighters, EMTs, paramedics, and construction workers. Yeah, we were guided by the spirit of a Lady in the harbor.

After a long shower, I sat with a can of Sapporo beer, exhausted and numb. As the cool beer went down my parched, hoarse throat, I suddenly saw the Blessed Mother. Hands were outstretched to her side. Below were the remnants of the Twin Towers. She was crying. Tears softly fell on the site and people there. I watched, unable to cry, unable to muster any emotion.

The following day, I called the academy to see if they needed me. The facility had been designated as a contact point for the families of the missing firemen. No one as of yet spoke of EMS losses. There would only be whispers and rumors for several weeks. The secretary answered the phone. I asked, "Do you need any volunteers?"

"Are you a fireman?"

"No. I'm a paramedic."

"Then call your battalion or somewhere, but not here."

The phone went dead.

Next, I called the Bureau of Health Services (BHS), where we give notification when we are taking a sick day.

"Sick Desk," the voice answered.

"Hello, I'm calling for a day." I needed it to get rid of this numbing, yet empty strangulation hold that enveloped me.

"Are you a fireman?"

"No, a paramedic. My cousin was killed on Rescue Three, and I spent seventeen hours there yesterday. I need the day."

Once again, "Are you a fireman?"

"No, a paramedic."

"Sorry, if you want off, you will have to come down and talk to a doctor who will decide if you get off or not."

I hung up the phone. Fuck the fire department. I was walking into walls and now I'm going down to see some scam artist FD doctor who will decide how I feel? Fuck them.

I reported in for my regular tour. Lieutenants Denise Werner and Giuseppe Lavore showed real concern, as did the crews at Battalion Twenty-six, when they heard about my cousin.

We were solemn as the TV screamed the latest reports. On the wall were pictures of the firefighters, and private reflections of our losses as the names started to drift in.

I had to do something. America, New York City, had been attacked.

My cousin, brothers and sister were murdered. Numerous of our EMTs were wounded, never waning in their efforts to save the victims.

Getting up off the couch, I walked to the phone. Once I had the number, I called.

"Excuse me!" Everyone looked. "Turn the TV down, please."

Suddenly everyone watched and listened. They had been concerned about me. But now I was on a mission.

A female answered the phone. "Afghanistan Mission, how might I help you?"

"Salom alakum," I said. The room got so quiet you could hear a pin drop.

Surprised and sounding very pleased, the woman returned the greeting.

Now that her defenses were down and before she could ask, I suckered her a little more.

"My name is Jim Schrang. That's Jim S-C-H-R-A-N-G."

Sounding like a dear friend, she responded, "Yes, Jim Schrang, and how can I help you?"

"Well, Madam. I am a New York City Fire Department paramedic, shield 3257, assigned to Battalion Twenty-six. I am also a Vietnam veteran who served with the One Hundred First Airborne Division, Screaming Eagles, in Vietnam."

"Yes," she responded in an inquiring, non-hostile voice.

"Madam, I have some good news and bad news for you."

"Good, bad news?"

"Yes, madam. The good news is I am praying and will continue to pray for your people and nation."

"Oh, thank you!" she responded in a cheery voice. "And the bad news, Jim?"

"The bad news is that after attacking America, you people are in deep shit."

She started cursing me in English, going into her own language, back to English. As the cursing continued, I said very calmly; "You have a mighty fine New York City EMS Day."

Hanging up, I turned around. Everyone just looked at me.

"Now I feel better. First shot in for America. Fuck them!" My ego felt great, not my spirit.

Suddenly the crew members' silence broke with, "Holy shit!" They started applauding. NYFD EMS had spoken. I felt like a ten-ton weight had been taken off my chest.

Upon hearing about the incident, Lieutenant Mercado stated his concern that they may have misunderstood what I said. His politically correct concern was that the Afghan Mission might construe it as a bomb threat. The fire department's BIT (Bureau of Investigation and Trials) might have to bring me up on charges.

I made my typical warm response, "Hey Rick, fuck them, the fire department, and you." One of the paramedics chimed in. "Hey, I don't think there was any misunderstanding. We all understood it clearly."

"Besides," chimed in an EMT, "Jim spelled out his name and where he is from in case they want to ask him in person."

This scared the shit out of the dear officer, who headed back to his desk. He was not too happy, since his office is by the front door.

One EMT looked at me. "You sure have some balls on you, I mean giving them name, shield, and address."

My response being my warm cuddly self: "Fuck them. We're Americans. And this is now an American fight."

Observations:

1. Command and Control -- such as it was -- was so completely disorganized on the organizational level such as FDNY, or EMS that it was nonexistent. Anything resembling cool-headed assessment of this catastrophic situation was only accomplished by ordinary individual members of EMS, PD, FD, and civilians in a living hell doing the extraordinary.

2. Why did NYPD set up their command post away from the building not in the lobby? Why did Ada Dolch, Principal of Leadership and Public High School a block from ground zero decide not to send her 600 kids into the lobby of the World Trade where the plan had stated they should be but decided to

evacuate the children to Battery Park where they were saved by hero ferry captains and crews? NYPD, knew it, Ada Dolch knew it, why didn't the 'experts' of FDNY know not to stage in and around the building?

3. FDNY brass never hesitated to send people into danger, repeatedly ordering people to do things that their own exercises, one a year prior and directives had shown them were not safe, not smart, and not how a professional, cutting edge segment of the Trinity of Emergency Services (PD, FDNY, and at the base EMS) would do the job. EMS administration without autonomy as the base of the Trinity, led by inept bureaucrats like Charlie Wells and Mark Stone followed willingly insuring ultimate failure and death while appeasing FDNY's ego.

4. "FDNY experts" becomes in this situation an oxymoron. FDNY Commissioner Von Essen's word, at this point, is worth less than the toilet paper you wipe your ass with. Giuliani's disastrous decisions regarding funding, organizational structure, political sellout, and overall destruction of EMS disqualifies him of any relevant "expert opinion." The fact is these two money mongering, non visionaries are the exact people who made those decisions to gut the system's preparedness. Thus just like the federal government deflecting blame concerning hurricane Katrina for FEMA's impotent criminal response; Von Essen and Giuliani would deflect blame by wrapping themselves in the American flag and using the emotions of a traumatized country and world to negate admitting their part in failure.

5. Calls from people who COULDN'T GET TO THE ROOF means that they were trying to do so. Sensitive equipment on the roof, security, is not an

excuse. It's a failure of planning from the architects, Port Authority side, not even mentioning **FDNY's ego which sealed not only the doors but 1,974 lives above the fire**. They had 8 years to figure it out folks from the first bombing. They didn't because they didn't care.

6. With one tower down it should have been OBVIOUS under the "Reasonable Man" theory (A standard that compares what a person with the same level of training would have done) and common sense that *ANY* attempt to help those people was worth it. Instead of going balls to the wall to save anyone sheer incompetence got far more people murdered than might have died during rescue attempts. "A few dozen people or even one" is a lot more than none, and to reiterate, those NYPD and military chopper pilots are the experts concerning extraction. **Chief of Department Peter J. Ganci, did in fact not employ all the resources he had on hand to save lives which he had taken an oath to do.** This is affirmed by the 9-11 Commission reports that though in FDNY and NYPD protocols for high-rise fires," No FDNY personnel were placed in NYPD helicopters." Further in the report, "...the FDNY Chief of Department had already *dismissed* any rooftop rescue as impossible."

7. **Looking deeper** into who the hell are these experts in FDNY , one needs to ask what are their credentials to give them such standing aside from wearing a firefighters uniform? What do those credentials mean in a world beyond that of one city's politics? Who hired them? Why? If we are to survive as a city and nation we need qualified leaders, not political and bar room, or in the current FDNY firehouse environment steroid, or cocaine pals. Another classic example of this is the current chief of FEMA Michael Brown.

Appointed by President Bush his last job was enforcing rules concerning breeding Arabian horses! Then people wonder why the national disgrace of hurricane Katrina and the murders of 9-11.

8. Walt Disney Productions offered "Everyone" that was at 9-11 one week free at Disney Land. When crews from hospitals like NY Cornell or St. Clare's called in they were curtly told "It's only for FDNY." Local 1199 and the Greater NY Hospital Fund found out about it and launched an investigation. By thy way if we check into who went from FDNY you'll find people who were not even at 9-11. **Only FDNY would and could spoil Disneyland** with their callous ignorance of separation. They weren't happy enough that they toured the world whining and covering up their failures at 9-11. No 'voluntary' hospital crews went on that trip either.

Rivalry, jealousy, greed, etc. all I claim is "Res ipsa Loquitor"—it speaks for itself.

Concerning taboo questions:
• Why, in 2001, if they are experts in fighting fires were New York's Bravest still climbing stairs in high-rises to fight fires?
• Why was my cousin murdered carrying a water hose when there was no water around, no super tanker to pressure it anyway, and it always takes foam to put out a jet-fuel fire?
• Why were there not fire department supply points on certain floors in high-rises?
• What was a seventy-year-old from another administration doing in uniform at a fire?
• Why were EMTs and paramedics ordered to pull their buses under the burning building? Why was Captain Mark Stone promoted and why does he and chief Charlie Wells still have their jobs?

• Why did you, Commissioner Von Essen, have officials from BITS sitting in on hearings concerning 9/11/01? Was he looking for scapegoats to deflect attention from yourself and Giuliani once Americans' public emotions calmed down and they asked for facts? Facts FDNY firefighters are still afraid to ask? I guess you and the Law and Order Mayor believed Lenin when he wrote, *"A lie told often enough becomes the truth."*

Finally, as the fires continued to rage at 'the pile' a statement came concerning EMS losses. On September 18, 2001, our union came out with a list. The union had been mute when the Fire God raged about the loss of over three hundred members, including my cousin, Jerry Schrang. This is our same union that watched silently as a police officer and a fireman stood before the president of the United States. No one represented EMS.

This silent, shameful leadership of local 2507 came up with the following breakdown, on a plain piece of white paper, never putting a name to the statistic.

EMS Injured: 116
FDEMS: 65
"Others": 51
EMS Missing:
FDEMS: 2
Voluntary Hospitals: 7
Private Ambulance: 1

We lost nine brothers and a sister. Yet the chiefs hid it. The union was dead silent about it. The only names that counted were firemen. Even our two FDNY paramedics are not even mentioned in the FD Museum today.

Eleven
And So It Goes

On October 2, 2001 EMT Sasha Gomez ran into the lounge area yelling that there was a fire in the apartment one building away from our facility at One Hundred Sixty-eighth Street and Boston Road in the South Bronx.

Paramedics Barry Goldberg, Neil Sweeting, and Joe Jefferson ran out. Joe was still on light duty assignment after being hurt at the World Trade Center. I went to my vehicle, grabbing the trauma bag, figuring someone might need to be intubated.

Outside the building, the local neighborhood people, junkies, and alcoholics, pointed to the second-floor window of the old, walk-up tenement. Colossal clouds of thick, gray-white smoke billowed from the window, quickly descending and obscuring the people and entrance.

People screamed as bright flames aggressively leapt from the exploding glass window frame. Four of New York's Finest had run into the building to see if anyone was in the apartment. The flames and heavy smoke forced two back. Barry, Mike, and Joe opted to try. After all, there were people still in this tinderbox, including two cops who might need help. Sasha ran to his locker, getting his helmet and turnout coat. Being new, he didn't want to get written up being out of uniform! Thus he was awarded the nickname, "Helmet Man."

Two cops huddled on the second floor in front of the blazing apartment. Suddenly, through the deadly smoke they saw blue uniforms and were heard to say, "Great, FD is here!" As the guys got closer they said, "Oh shit, it's EMS!" Talk about being loved.

After grabbing my bag, I approached the building. The people pointed to the building, as if I needed help in locating the now major fire. The hallway was totally obscured, as the gray-black smoke drifted out the lobby door. Running inside, I banged on doors, losing sight of the outside world. After locating the stairwell, I proceeded up, fighting the downward-rolling smoke.

"Does that fire extinguisher work?" I heard Barry ask, from somewhere above me.

"Yeah."

"Then give it to me! You won't need it."

Seemed that the young male tenant, who passed me on the stairs, was trying to run out of a burning building with a fully charged fire extinguisher!

Like Barry said, "You won't need it."

At the first landing I found Neil, arguing with an overweight, obnoxious, elderly African- American female. We had all come to know and despise her because of needless 911 calls. She was on the phone talking, as the apartment next door was afire.

Joe said, "Please hang up."

She responded, "But I'm not done talking."

With this, Joe took the phone, after a slight struggle, and hung it up.

"But I want to call my husband," she yelled as they dragged the overweight heifer beast into the hallway. Unfortunately, they were dragging her on a very old wooden kitchen chair. I could hear the guys, as well as the chair, groaning.

Barry was at the fire door. He had attempted to rush into the apartment to do a search, but was forced back by the flames. He was kneeling, keeping the door slightly open.

"I've got to keep this open for the engine company!" he yelled over the crackling sound of the flames destroying all within and the heifer bitching she couldn't now breathe!

Barry is a volunteer fireman in Long Island, so I guess the reason for keeping the door open was so the firemen could find the fire. Hey, there was a lot of smoke. Seriously though, I trusted him with all our lives.

I squatted next to him. We heard movement. Looking over our shoulder through the dense smoke, we saw Neil, Joe, and Sasha. They were dragging the old wooden chair closer to the staircase. Once at the stairs, they cursed and yelled to someone below, "We need one of our chairs. She's too big!" Talk about understatements.

Paramedic Lorna "Cookie" O'Farrell, who was on light duty while recovering from an operation, came running. For normal people it would be walking. But since she and Bubba are about the same height, well, you get the picture.

She remembered there was an elderly gentleman in the building who was hearing-impaired. Thus when alerted of the fire, Cookie took it upon herself and entered the building. Groping in the acrid smoke, banging on the elderly man's door, she but heard the call for a chair, ran back to the garage and got one. There were only two problems. First, Cookie is short as stated, so it took a few minutes for her to cover the distance. Thus, Neil, Joe, and Sasha were motivated by the flames, increasing heat and life-choking smoke not to wait.

They figured the better part of valor was to duff the area, fast. Especially since the old wooden staircase was the only way out. They went down the stairs, almost literally, in the blinding smoke, with the now combative heifer. Once in the lobby, they continued to drag the chair until they saw Cookie.

Cookie could get an asthma attack just from walking. She has been intubated several times. Yet, being a true Street Saint of Compassion, she answered the call and put herself second to the care of others.

"Is everybody out from upstairs?" I asked Barry.

"I don't know."

"Okay, I'm going up." I started climbing up the stairs.

"I'll cover you with the fire extinguisher." At that moment, the two cops appeared. They had been below the chair with the beast in it and saw the crew members struggling. They decided to take their chances against the flames instead of attempting to lift her. Up we went, banging on doors. And down we came with the cops in the lead.

One tenant was behind me, arguing.

"I don't need to leave no place."

"Shut the fuck up and get out of here, now!" I yelled.

"You heard my partner," Barry said as he stood up.

This fool continued down the stairs, smoking his cigarette.

At this point I was coughing up my lungs.

"Go downstairs, Jim," Barry said.

"I will not leave my wing man, I mean partner."

With this we were both hysterical choking, gagging and laughing tears filling our eyes.

"Wrong movie," I said, gasping for air.

"Yeah…"

Looking down the stairwell a police sergeant with two officers ordering an evacuation.

"I'm ordering you out of this building!" he yelled.

Just then one of the Bravest entered with a water hose and of course no Scott pack on either his back or face. Boy was I glad to see him.

"Barry, let's get out. FD is here."

I still don't understand it, but Barry beat me out of the building. Once outside, he saw Neil down on one knee, holding his side.

"Are you okay?"

"It's my side. I think I pulled a muscle," Neil moaned in agony.

"Okay, can you make it to the garage?"

"I'll try, check on Cookie."

Someone had placed a radio call that EMS crews were trapped in a burning building. Upon hearing this, crews started to "buff" the job.

Barry spotted Cookie on all fours, gasping for air. He and several other crew members from responding units grabbed her. Plopping her into the stair chair, they rushed toward the garage out of the pungent, smoky, diesel-fumed environment as more engines and buses continued to respond in.

Joe asked the old lady, "Are you okay?" as she breathed through an oxygen mask.

"Yes. Could you please go upstairs and get my purse?"

Joe, who in his own right is mellow, looked up to heaven. But heaven was blocked as the other windows exploded. Searing flames and smoke continued to belch forth. With an EMT there, Joe quietly walked away as the woman continued to complain about her purse.

During this time, Lieutenant Juan Correa had been on the phone alerting, requesting, and coordinating the responding resources. Aside from this, he kept the tour commander advised of the situation. If it weren't for him, it would have been a hurting situation. Over the last several months under the tutelage of Captain Andy Werner and Deputy Chief Carl Tramontana, Correa had done a one hundred-and-eighty–degree turn. His new attitude and concern were reflected in his timely, professional handling of this near-tragic event.

Stumbling out of the lobby, I went to a Basic unit for some oxygen, my lungs burning.

"How is everybody?" I gasped, coughing uncontrollably as one of the crew members treated a civilian.

"Cookie is in bad shape. They dragged her into the office. Hey, where are you . . ."

Before he could finish, I got out and ran to the office with my drug bag, realizing she might need to be tubed again. Upon entering the office, I found Lieutenant Correa with numerous units assisting. Cookie was really tight, so Correa decided to take us all to Jacobi Hospital, where they have the hyperbaric chamber if we needed it. I didn't want to go, but Lieutenant Correa would not hear otherwise.

Before we got to Jacobi, we were told our Division Commander, Frances Pascale (nicknamed Old Knee Pads...) was giving Lieutenant Correa a hard time. She didn't like the fact that he "allowed and didn't stop" us from entering the burning building. The term "out of job title" was used to describe our actions. This, from a person who freaked at ground zero tying up essential units who wore a white paramedic patch but was another Mark Stone, not a real street paramedic but a 'pass the written test every 3 years' medic.

Once at Jacobi, the fun started. Staff took our vital signs as we sucked oxygen and filled out the registration information. One fireman, who had been slightly hurt, sat across from us. On the form, everyone except me placed 9 Metro Tech as the home address. I told the guys not to, but they did. Later the woman from registration came out and had them correct the paperwork. She explained, "Only firemen can use 9 Metro Tech."

"Gee, I don't understand that," stated EMS Command Chief Robert McCracken to Chief Basile (The snake), EMS Division 5 Commander.

"Because we are civilian employees, thanks to you," I muttered under my breath. It got a chuckle from Barry, sitting near me.

At that point, Chief Pascale looked directly at me and gleefully announced,

"The fire department battalion chief said you all did a fantastic job. So I want you to write yourselves up so you can get awards!"

"Not in your life," I said.

She ignored me.

"Oh, what you guys need are resuscitators," she said.

"What we need are gas masks," I retorted adamantly.

Now frantically looking around to exit the area, she exclaimed,

"Where's Cookie? I must see Cookie!" With that, she was gone.

"Jim, did I hear you are leaving in January?" McCracken asked.

"Yeah," I answered, closing my eyes. I was doing yoga breathing since my blood pressure was up when I had the initial set of vitals taken. I knew I could lower my blood pressure.

"Let me know."

"Not in your life," I closed my eyes again.

He looked at Vice President Don Faeth of our local, standing next to him. Don has known me for many years and knew McCracken should have just let it die there.

"Why are you leaving?"

"After what you did to us at the World Trade Center, you have to ask?"

This time I stared at him. He was totally blown away, but still in the politically correct ass wipe Fire God mode. He actually grabbed my hand and yelled, "I don't have to take this. Goodbye!"

Don, realizing I was on a rip, remembered he was late for a meeting and left... fast!

Barry decided to go see how Cookie was doing. I was left with Captain Jerry Gelbard who was helping with the paperwork. Jerry was the commanding officer for Battalion Fourteen at Lincoln Hospital and a good guy.

As for Cookie, I realized she was fine as she kept making silly faces at us from the nice hospital bed. Typical woman! She got the soft bed, while we got the hard plastic chairs.

"Dario is 10-9," Jerry said. This meant the good Dr. Dario Gonzalez was at the hospital.

"I'm going to take a piss," I said to a laughing Jerry. He knew very well how the troops, and I in particular, felt about the infamous doctor.

Upon my return, Dario was with Cookie. I stood with Barry and Jerry. My blood pressure came down just as I said it would, as I joked with a nurse who marveled at the results of a few minutes of meditation. Dario walked over and slapped Barry on the shoulder, saying, "Nice job. Feel better." Then walked out, never even acknowledging my existence. Barry, with embarrassing shock written all over his face, looked at the now hysterical captain.

"He knew better than to even open his mouth to you." Jerry said, placing his arm around me through the laughter.

"Yeah, but that was rude. He never even looked you in the eyes, Jim," Barry said, still shocked.

"He knew better. He knows, that I know, what he and the rest of them are. Anybody hungry?" I asked. Well they do have a McDonald's at Jacobi Hospital, ah American healthcare.

It turned out to be a good day, and a great way to finish my career at FDNY EMS.

Epilogue

Over the last few years FDNY has demanded to have a "separate" memorial, ad nauseam. If there was a camera, there was a firefighter in his bunker coat demonstrating a bunker mentality, whining for a separate memorial. My personal opinion is that their ego brings dishonor to all of us.

On that day, there were basically three types of people. There were the terrorists who lived and died by hatred, believing in "Our god is greater than yours!" Next, we had the victims who went to work that morning thinking of their families, jobs, and other things. Finally, there were all of us who responded, not seeing any difference in anyone, but rather seeing people hurt and dying. The planes exploded with the deafening roar of man-made hatred. Their flaming wreckage appeared as bright as rockets slicing deeply into Mother Earth and searing open the very gates of man's insane belief of separation.

In that moment, a family of American civilian EMTs and paramedics stood, never yielding. They fought, and died shoulder to shoulder along with New York City's Bravest and Finest, PA police, and others who were of one conscience, one belief—love. In the searing flames of man's inhumanity to man blossomed a garden of sacred flowers, nourished by blood, sweat, and tears. Each petal represented one of these noble people, not just us, but the victims also. Each one of us served in a noble profession. EMTs and paramedics were peaceful healers, yet true warriors not taking lives, giving our all so others might live. Each a true "Currahee." We "Stand Alone," rose above the insanity and hatred, realizing, as I believe the victims knew on a higher consciousness, that they, as well as our fallen brothers and sister, were there to teach a sacred lesson.

Not one victim, not one rescuer, not even the insane terrorists, died in vain. Only if we honor the terrorists' belief of separation, and superiority, do we fail to learn the lesson.

Thus, I would like to see one monument with the names of everyone in alphabetical order, under or next to each name the country they hailed from. As for the rescuers, intermingle their names like the points of loving beams of hope they were that day, with their department or title under their names forming a mosaic of love. In this way when children such as Yamel's son visit the site, they will need to actively search through thousands of names to find their dad or mom. It will allow Yamel's son, for instance, to see all the people Yamel, her brother and sister EMTs and paramedics, as well as firefighters and police officers touched that day in love. It is a way of gently planting a seed of love more powerful than a separate, isolated egotistical concrete memorial.

When the fires of hatred and insanity devoured thousands of innocents, these healers paid the ultimate price to keep the flame of eternal love alive, searing the hatred away.

On May 24, 2007 there was the Memorial run to the World Trade Center. That day 150 U.S. Marines from the USS Wasp proudly led NYPD and FDNY on the run. Not one member of EMS was invited.

Yamel Merino, EMT
MetroCare Ambulance

Keith Fairben, Mario Santoro, Paramedics New York
Presbyterian New York Presbyterian

Richard Quinn, Carlos Lillo, Paramedics FDNY EMS
Battalion 57 FDNY EMS Battalion 49

Mark Schwartz, Richard Allen Pearlman, EMT's
Hunter Ambulance, Forest Hills Volunteer Ambulance

David Mark Sullins, EMT
Cabrini Hospital Medical Center

David P. Lemagne, Paramedic
Jersey City Medical Center Port Authority Police Officer

Mitch Wallace, EMT Bayside Volunteer Ambulance
Court Officer

Made in the USA
Monee, IL
07 July 2026

56550057R00167